D0907133

To Relieve the Human Condition

Bioethics, Technology, and the Body

Gerald P. McKenny

State University of New York Press

Published by
State University of New York Press, Albany

© 1997 State University of New York

For information, address State University of New York
Press, State University Plaza, Albany, N.Y. 12246

Production by E. Moore
Marketing by Bernadette LaManna

Library of Congress Cataloging-in-Publication Data

McKenny, Gerald P.
    To relieve the human condition : bioethics, technology, and the
  body / Gerald P. McKenny.
        p.   cm.
    Includes bibliographical references and index.
    ISBN 0-7914-3473-7 (hc : alk. paper). — ISBN 0-7914-3474-5 (pbk.
  : alk. paper)
    1. Medical ethics. 2. Bioethics. I. Title.
  R724.M2922 1997
  174′.2—dc20   96-45998
                                                              CIP

10 9 8 7 6 5 4 3 2 1

*To my mother
and the memory of my father*

Contents

Acknowledgments

This book would have been unthinkable without the insight and support of many people. I am indebted to two of my teachers, James Gustafson, who first led me to think of the issues I address here, and Robin Lovin, who taught me how to think about them philosophically. Additional debts are owed to colleagues at Rice University and the Texas Medical Center at Houston. H. Tristram Engelhardt, Jr., impressed on me the limits of standard forms of bioethical inquiry and the need for particular traditions to resolve most bioethical problems, while B. Andrew Lustig repeatedly led me to formulate more rigorously my positions on the particular bioethical issues I treat here. Werner Kelber, Anne Klein, and Edith Wyschogrod convinced me of the importance of the body as a central point of inquiry, while Stanley Reiser influenced my thinking about the role of technology in medicine. George Khushf and Allen Verhey were indispensible in helping me to think theologically about this project. William Parsons served as a sounding board for many of my ideas.

More specific debts are owed to the following persons: to Stanley Hauerwas, George Khushf, William Parsons, and several anonymous readers for SUNY Press for their helpful insights and comments on all or part of the manuscript; to H. Tristram Engelhardt, Jr., and Kai Hoshino for an invitation to present an earlier version of chapter one to the U.S.-Japan Bioethics Congress in Tokyo in 1994, and to Robert Veatch for his comments; to the faculty of the Institute for the Medical Humanities at the University of Texas Medical Branch at Galveston for inviting me to present an overview of this project at a faculty colloquium, during which I benefited from their insightful comments and persistent questions; and to the Dean of Humanities at Rice University for a semester leave during which I began work on this project. I am grateful to Martin Kavka for his work in preparing the index. Finally, I am indebted to Phimpmas, for her support and encouragement and for continually putting before me the question of why any of this is important.

In addition to these personal debts, I am grateful for permission to quote copyrighted materials from the following sources and publishers:

Ethics from a Theocentric Perspective, vol. 2, by James M. Gustafson, © 1984 by the University of Chicago Press;

The Imperative of Responsibility, by Hans Jonas, © 1984 by the University of Chicago Press;

Suffering Presence: Theological Reflections on Medicine, the Mentally Handicapped and the Church, by Stanley Hauerwas, © 1986 by the University of Notre Dame Press;

"Making Babies: The New Biology and the 'Old' Morality, by Leon Kass, © 1972 by *The Public Interest.*

I am also grateful for permission to reprint, as parts of chapters one and two, respectively, portions of the following previously published titles:

"Technology, Authority and the Loss of Tradition: The Roots of American Bioethics in Comparison with Japanese Bioethics," by Gerald P. McKenny, *Japanese and Western Bioethics: Studies in Moral Diversity*, edited by Kazumasa Hoshino, © 1997 Kluwer Academic Publishers, pp. 73–87. Reprinted by permission of Kluwer Academic Publishers.

"Physician-Assisted Death: A Pyrrhic Victory for Secular Bioethics," by Gerald P. McKenny, *Secular Bioethics in Theological Perspective*, edited by Earl E. Shelp, © 1996 Kluwer Academic Publishers, pp. 145–58. Reprinted by permission of Kluwer Academic Publishers.

Introduction

In Book III of the *Republic*, while discussing the training for the guardians of his ideal city, Plato addresses the role of medicine in their formation. His underlying question is how the pursuit of health can be so managed that medicine serves rather than hinders or dominates our moral projects. This question in turn breaks down into several more specific questions: How much attention or vigilance should we devote to our bodies in the effort to optimize their capacities? How much control should we allow physicians to exercise over our bodies? What ends, individual and collective, should determine what counts as a sufficiently healthy body? What limits should we observe in our efforts to improve our bodily performance and remove causes of suffering (Plato, 403c–407a)?

Ludwig Edelstein, the historian of ancient Greek medicine, reminds us of the context for these questions. Ancient physicians advocated the notion that without a high level of health no other goods are possible and that even the healthy should follow the dictates of physicians, which were comprehensive enough to require an almost continuous monitoring of one's bodily life. Fearing that to follow these dictates would make one a slave of the body and of one's physician, a major task of philosophers such as Plato was to oppose the glorification of health, the excessive vigilance it involved, and the underlying claim that health is the highest human good (Edelstein, 1967, pp. 357–359).

Had the term *bioethics* existed in Plato's time there is little doubt that the questions he raised would have constituted its agenda. Yet these questions are virtually absent from the mainstream agenda of the enterprise we call bioethics. This would perhaps be less of a problem if the analogies between the ancient Greek estimation of the pursuit of bodily perfection and our own were not so strong. But if the analogies are so strong, why has contemporary bioethics not taken up Plato's agenda? I shall argue that one reason is that our obsession with bodily perfection occurs under a moral imperative that originated with the rise of modern technology and that, in the writings of Francis Bacon and Rene Descartes, looks to medicine for its actualization. Modern medicine, with its immense capacities to intervene into and reorder the body, continually holds out the promise of fulfilling this imperative. The imperative is to eliminate suffering and to expand the realm of human choice—in short, to relieve the human condition of subjection to the whims of fortune or the bonds of natural necessity. The complicity of standard forms of bioethics in this Baconian project, as I call it, impoverishes bioethics in two ways. First, while relief of suffering and expansion of choice are laudable goals, standard bioethics provides no moral framework within which to determine what kinds of suffering should be eliminated and which choices are best. Medicine is therefore called on to eliminate whatever anyone might consider a burden of finitude. Second, standard bioethics is incapable of addressing moral implications of the way technological medicine constructs and controls the body. The result of this twofold impoverishment is that standard bioethics is silent on many of the most urgent moral questions raised by the technological transformation of medicine. These are the questions Plato raised: the attention or vigilance we should devote to the state of our bodily health relative to other matters, the degree of control over our bodies we should surrender to medicine, the individual and collective ends that determine what counts as adequate health, and the limits to improving our bodies and eliminating suffering.

The failure to address these and related questions cannot be overcome by a better bioethical theory of the standard variety. For such questions pose the problem of the place of the body—its health, its capacities, its susceptibility to illness and suffering, and its mortality—in a morally worthy life, and for reasons that will become clear in chapter one, standard forms of bioethics cannot address these issues. Accordingly, I argue that the task of bioethics is to explore the moral significance of the body as it is expressed in particular moral and religious traditions—a moral significance that is denied in the efforts of the Baconian project to rescue the body from fortune or necessity. This alternative agenda builds on (and criticizes) the work of theologians, philosophers, and physicians who have challenged what I will call the technological utopianism that characterizes the Baconian project, but who have heretofore been viewed as isolated critics rather than as part of a common endeavor. By presenting these diverse critics as neverthe-less united in opposition to the Baconian project, I place my alterna-tive agenda within an ongoing conversation and bring a new focus to a field whose novelty regarding the issues it addresses increasingly masks a stagnant uniformity in the methods and assumptions it brings to those issues.

The following chapters divide themselves into two parts. The first part, comprising the first two chapters, is a critique of standard bioethics. Chapter one traces standard bioethics to a moral discourse that replaced traditional ways of understanding the moral significance of the body, the pursuit of health, and the suffering connected with ill-ness. Far from constituting a rationally vindicated response to technol-ogy or to the need for a common morality, as its advocates claim, I argue that standard bioethics is rooted in this modern discourse that underwrites the Baconian project and prevents challenges to its tech-nological utopianism from being heard. Following this general critique, chapter two examines the issues of physician-assisted death and germ-line gene therapy to illustrate how standard bioethics is unable to answer many of the most urgent questions posed by the Baconian pro-ject.

The second part consists of detailed analyses of critics of the Baconian project and their alternatives to it. These criticisms and alter-natives fall under three headings: nature, tradition, and the body. The first two of these critics, Hans Jonas and James Gustafson, attempt to wrest from modern discourse about nature and morality a normative conception of the human. While both use some of the resources of mod-ern science and accept some of the limitations that modern secular thought imposes on such a conception, both find in modern discourses of nature (including human nature) and morality the sources of the technological utopianism of modern medicine. Jonas opposes the nihilism that results from the metaphysical neutralization of nature while Gustafson challenges the modern confidence that nature exists to serve human purposes. Chapters three and four examine their analyses of technological utopianism and their efforts to limit it by a normative conception of the human grounded in what each argues is a more ade-quate understanding of nature.

The next two critics turn to tradition to limit the Baconian ambi-tions of medicine. They wrestle with an ancient question: To what extent does medicine as a practice or profession constitute a self-sufficient moral tradition and to what extent does it require an account of the good from another source in order to achieve its telos or carry out its commitments? Chapter five examines the work of physician and humanistic scholar Leon Kass. Kass reformulates a traditional teleological conception of medicine as a practice, ultimately backed by a conception of human flourishing and supported by a broader order of institutions and practices, in which he finds a normative conception of health he believes is capable of determining the proper ends of medicine and the proper scope of its technological interventions. In contrast, theologian Stanley Hauerwas argues that only a particular religious community can supply the necessary understanding of the good and the practices that embody it. Hence only such a community can sustain medicine as a traditional practice against the technological ambitions and pretensions nourished by a liberal society. Chapter six describes how for Hauerwas the Christian church and its practices of reconciliation serve as a contrast model to such a society and a form of resistance to the Baconian project.

While ideas of embodiment are central in the accounts of Jonas and Kass, the final set of critics turn to the ways in which the body is constructed and controlled by modern medicine. Chapter seven explores the analyses of technological control of the body carried out by phenomenologists Drew Leder and Richard Zaner and by critical theorist Michel Foucault. All three show how the mechanistic view of the body that developed between the seventeenth and early nineteenth centuries brought questions of the meaning of the body, its mortality, and its susceptibility to illness under the domain of medicine with its increasing technological prowess. In addition, Foucault's analyses of biopower show how control over the body is disseminated through various social and administrative networks and operates through the production of forms of knowledge about the body and the stimulation of desires for a certain kind of body. Using feminist perspectives on the body as a bridge between phenomenology and critical theory, I show how expansion of choice and the desire to eliminate suffering enable society through the offices of technological medicine to produce the kinds of bodies it needs. Foucault's analyses strike at the heart of the Baconian project, namely, its claim to have expanded human freedom.

My approach in these chapters is analytical and critical: I examine each position as an alternative to the Baconian project and identify its shortcomings. These chapters therefore serve as critical surveys of important bioethicists vis-à-vis Baconian medicine and can be used as such. But my evaluations at the end of each chapter are constructive. They point to the position I defend in chapter eight: that the utopian effort to render our lives free from fate or fortune has impoverished our moral lives and entangled us in new forms of control, and that consequently a recovery of the moral significance of the body is necessary.

After a summary of the three types of alternative to the Baconian project, I illustrate in chapter eight the kind of inquiry I believe bioethics should pursue by briefly examining how the view of the moral significance of the body in Christianity answers Plato's questions. The premise of my constructive task is that moral subjects are formed and form themselves in part by interpreting and acting on their bodies. If I am right, then medicine in this technological era plays an important role in forming us as moral subjects, and a major task of bioethics is to determine what this role should be. This chapter not only provides a new locus for questions about technology and ethics but also calls attention to the importance for religious ethics more generally of questions about the significance of the body for morality and of morality for the body.

Some explanations of certain aspects of what follows are in order. The first concerns my term "technological utopianism." First, I believe medicine has always been technological in the sense that it has always sought more effectual ways to intervene into and reorder bodily processes. Since this intervention into and reordering of the body is my criterion of technology, I (like James Gustafson) take the distinctive mark of *modern* technology to be the vastly expanded scope of such intervention and reordering rather than, say, its artificiality (Hans Jonas) or its devices (Albert Borgmann and Stanley Reiser), however significant I believe these other criteria are for a fuller understanding of modern technology. Second, while I agree with Daniel Callahan that modern medicine is not utopian in the sense that it offers a detailed plan for where technology ought to take us, I also agree with Jonas that a chief characteristic of modern utopia is that no such plan is needed. To the extent that the task of medicine is to continue indefinitely to expand our choices and eliminate suffering and thus to relieve our subjection to fortune and finitude, it is justifiably viewed as utopian.

A second point is related to the first. Nothing that follows warrants the designation of this work as antitechnology or antimedicine. To the contrary, I express doubts about those views that would reduce our alternatives to standing over against technology or being swallowed up by it, and argue instead for appropriating technology as well as resisting it. The problem is not technology itself but our lack of a moral framework that can tell us how rightly to resist and appropriate it. Similarly, I do not argue against medicine or even its current technological focus, but rather defend a more limited role for medicine as currently practiced. Medicine in my scheme would find its place as one part (and not always the most important part) of a much broader practice of care, itself grounded in a view of the moral significance of the body.

The third matter requiring explanation is my choice of authors with and against whom to work out my position. Obviously other choices could have been made. Among the theologians, I chose Gustafson and Hauerwas because they have dealt more explicity with the Baconian project than have Germain Grisez, Richard McCormick, and Paul Ramsey, all of whom I seriously considered. Among philosophically minded critics, Daniel Callahan has persistently raised the issues I address here over a quarter of a century, but I finally decided on Leon Kass because the latter has developed his position in view of the questions about the body that I have found so significant for dealing with these issues. Similarly, among phenomenologists and critical theorists I chose Drew Leder, Richard Zaner, and Michel Foucault over thinkers such as Donna Haraway and Iris Marion Young because of their greater attention to the analysis of Baconian medicine.

CHAPTER 1

Technology, Tradition,
and the Origins of Bioethics

When the issues we now call bioethical first captured public attention more than a quarter century ago, far-reaching developments were already changing the way we give and receive medical care. These changes were rooted in the capacity of medicine to intervene into natural processes such that vast areas of life once subject to natural necessity or fate now became susceptible to human intervention. The effects wrought by this power to intervene are monumental, pervasive and apparently irreversible. They include the extension of medical authority over new areas of our lives, the expansion of technological control of the body, the transformation of questions about the place of illness and health in a morally worthy life into questions about which preferences technology should fulfil, the implications of pursuing the Enlightenment hope of a progressive elimination of pain and suffering from human life. These and other effects raise profound moral questions about the proper extent of the power of medicine over our lives, the moral and social limits of technological interventions, and the individual and social ends that the pursuit of health should serve.

The authors I discuss in this volume have devoted most of their work in bioethics to addressing questions such as these. Yet their preoccupations have been ignored by most mainstream bioethicists, whose own writings have remained strangely silent on these and related questions. The silence is strange because some of the most pressing problems bioethics currently faces—including the question of how to set limits on health care costs and the potential uses and abuses of genetic technology—seem to require reflection on the proper scope and limits of the technological transformation of medicine. My ultimate aim in this volume is to overcome this silence by putting such questions on the agenda of bioethics. But in order to accomplish this I must first understand the reasons for it. The silence is lamentable but on reflection not surprising. Standard bioethics, by which I mean the family of secular approaches rooted in the theories and principles of analytical moral philosophy that are dominant in the English-speaking world, is a product of modernity, and the moral task of modernity is to resolve conflicts between competing interests in order to secure social cooperation without appeal to robust views of the good. The agenda of standard bioethics, at the risk of oversimplification, follows accordingly: for every new issue that arises in biomedical research and care its task is to safeguard individual autonomy, calculate potential risks and harms, and determine whether or not a just distribution will follow. It would be foolish to deny the importance of this agenda.[1] Nevertheless, one blissfully ignorant of moral philosophy might wonder what the silence regarding the moral implications of the technological transformation of medicine would say if it were allowed to speak. Does it simply reflect the narrowness of modern moral theories, which eschew questions that seem to fall within the domain of sociology or religion? Or does it indicate a suppression of questions that challenge a deep but implicit moral agreement between standard bioethics and the effort to overcome the human subjection to fate or natural necessity?

In order to challenge standard bioethics in this way, it is not sufficient to argue that bioethicists fail to justify their basic principles or conclusions, since such a failure in execution need not implicate the agenda itself. Instead, this type of challenge requires a more fundamental inquiry into what accounts for the kinds of questions standard bioethics raises about the contemporary practice of medicine, the range of concerns it addresses, and the moral issues it believes are at stake. The pursuit of these questions calls for a certain kind of hermeneutical investigation—one that, in Charles Taylor's terms, seeks to understand the appeal of a cultural phenomenon by supplying "an interpretation . . . which will show why people found (or find) it convincing/inspiring/moving, which will identify what can be called the 'idees-forces' it contains" (Taylor, 1989, p. 202). This kind of interpretation identifies the moral sources which constitute the attractiveness or worthiness of the moral vision to those who adhere to it by constructing a narrative account of the origins and development of these sources. In this chapter I adapt (somewhat loosely) both the method and (with considerable modifications) the results of Taylor's investigation in order to articulate the moral sources of standard bioethics and of modern technological medicine. These sources, I argue, include moral convictions about the importance of the relief of suffering and the expansion of human choice. These convictions are deeply intertwined with religious and secular beliefs about nature and attitudes and practices regarding the body. Together these convictions, beliefs, attitudes and practices constitute a transvaluation of traditional values regarding the body and the pursuit of health. In brief, a moral discourse that related the health of the body as well as its mortality and its susceptibility to illness and suffering to broader conceptions of a morally worthy life was succeeded by a moral discourse characterized by efforts to eliminate suffering and expand human choice and thereby overcome the human subjection to natural necessity or fate. The result is that standard bioethics moves within the orbit of the technological utopianism of what I call the Baconian project (my term for the new discourse and the set of practices in which it is embedded), and its agenda and content are designed to resolve certain issues and problems that arise within that project.

A hermeneutical account of this sort is designed to answer the question of what makes a moral framework or discourse worthy of adherence among those committed to it.[2] But because of their function, such accounts (Taylor's included) use the past in order to render the agent's current moral self-understanding more secure and to confirm the agent in his or her moral identity. Hence while a hermeneutical account is necessary to articulate the moral sources of standard bioethics, it alone is not sufficient to call the moral identity of the latter into question. It must therefore be corrected and supplemented by an adaptation of the type of archealogical account that Michel Foucault specialized in (Foucault, 1972).[3] The archealogical task is to show how a cultural phenomenon is limited by the range of concepts, objects, norms of reasoning, and so on that comprise its realm of discourse. Standard bioethics, from this perspective, participates in a discursive formation in which, for example, traditional ways of conceptualizing and objectifying the body in relation to moral ends and authorities were radically altered or replaced altogether. Hence the newer discourse could no longer artic-ulate the moral insights and concerns of the earlier discourse, which were forgotten, distorted or rejected. This kind of inquiry is important as a correction or supplement to a hermeneutical inquiry because it shows how questions central to premodern traditions as well as more recent questions regarding the Baconian project itself will be marginalized or ignored in standard bioethics. Hence the silence regarding questions such as those I identified above.[4]

Taylor's hermeneutical method and Foucault's archealogical method both require inquiry into the origins of moral discourses. The field of bioethics is, relatively speaking, still in its youth, and like most youths it is unburdened by propensities to reflect on its origins. Nevertheless, those bioethicists who have engaged in such reflection have tended to narrate two accounts of the origin of their field. Both accounts find the origins of bioethics in cultural problems that allegedly require the types of solutions standard bioethics offers. One account refers to the need for solutions to the quandaries presented by modern technology, while the other refers to the need for a common morality to resolve a crisis of moral authority. It is, of course, in the interests of standard bioethicists to find the origins of their movement in these cultural needs. If technology presents moral problems that standard bioethics alone can resolve or if standard bioethics can claim a public moral authority that traditional moral schemes have lost, then as long as technology and contested moral authority are inevitable features of our culture, the agenda of standard bioethics—the questions, range of concerns, and moral issues it addresses—would be rationally vindicated.

I begin, therefore, by showing how technology does not require standard bioethics and how the latter obscures what is at issue in the crisis of moral authority, namely why the agenda of standard bioethics is still plausible despite its failure to resolve the crisis of moral authority. This leads to my alternative account which traces the agenda of standard bioethics to a moral discourse that excludes, marginalizes, or distorts the questions and concerns I alluded to in the opening paragraph. I provide in this chapter only a sketch of this discourse, which is developed further through authors treated in later chapters. But if I succeed here in showing how standard bioethics arises in a contingent and limited discourse, it then becomes possible to imagine a bioethical agenda constructed around other questions—questions such as those Plato raised, which concern the proper place of the technological control of the body in the moral lives of persons and communities. I believe that my account is rationally superior to those narrated by standard bioethicists; that is, I believe I give a more adequate account of the agenda of bioethics and the self-evident plausibility it has for many modern persons.[5] But in addition to giving what I believe is a more adequate account, my venture will succeed if it rescues from the margins a group of thinkers whose questions are as vital to the health of bioethics as they are absent from its current diet.

BIOETHICS AND THE RISE OF TECHNOLOGY

Bioethicists trained in moral philosophy often assume that their field of study is the product of the remarkable technological developments of recent decades that have irrevocably changed the way medicine is practiced. In its simplest form, this argument appeals to the moral quandaries of modern technological medicine which, because they are believed to be unprecedented, render traditional medical and religious ethical systems obsolete. Technology, so the argument goes, has made it possible to intervene into natural processes in ways these religious and medical traditions never anticipated, producing moral dilemmas which they are incapable of resolving. As a result we are forced to make moral choices about matters on which they can provide no guidance. A new, philosophically grounded bioethics is therefore necessary. Now that there is such a bioethics, religious and medical traditions can be dismissed as relics of the past, to be replaced by the application of common moral principles or casuistical techniques to these unprecedented problems.

This is a familiar way for bioethicists, physicians, lawyers, and policy experts to account for the origins of bioethics (Emanuel, 1991, pp. 9–14). But I believe it is mistaken. Why it is mistaken can be illustrated with reference to an event frequently mentioned in support of this view: the 1968 declaration on brain death by the Ad Hoc Committee of the Harvard Medical School to Examine the Definition of Death. The declaration was a response to moral difficulties occasioned by the capacity to sustain respiratory functions by mechanical ventilation and thus seems to supply a paradigm instance of technology creating an unprecendented problem requiring a novel solution. But the declaration and its place in the ongoing debate on brain death also provide evidence against this assumption. First, however novel are the problems posed by new technology, they are not always entirely unprecedented. Concern about how to define death has a long history in medicine (Lock and Honde, 1990) and in many religious traditions, and the same is true of many other "unprecedented" issues. Second, religious and medical traditions are just as capable of extending traditional insights to the new problems posed by technological medicine as they were when faced by the economic and political changes that accompanied the modern era. Some of these traditions, including rabbinic Judaism, have arrived at positions on brain death without using the principles or methods of secular bioethics (Bleich, 1989; Jakobovits, 1989). Third, as indicated by the continuing controversies over brain death and by the differences in the way brain death has been received in the United States and Japan, it is often impossible to generate moral principles and apply them to cases without involving oneself in deeply held cultural or religious beliefs and practices (Zaner, 1988a; Lock and Honde, 1990).

If the issue of brain death is representative, as I believe it is, then the moral dilemmas generated by new medical technology do not account for the moral appeal of standard bioethics nor rationally vindicate its agenda or content. The growth of new technology can not account for the attractiveness or worthiness of standard bioethics or justify its agenda.

BIOETHICS AND THE
CRISIS OF MORAL AUTHORITY

Of course, technology has been a determinative factor—perhaps the most determinative factor—in the practice of medicine over the past two centuries and especially the past half century. Indeed my argument below assumes the prominence of technology and points to an intimate relationship between standard bioethics and technology. But at this point I have argued only that the reign of technology, as Stanley Reiser calls it, does not require the reign of standard bioethics. Yet if technology itself does not require standard bioethics, one may ask how within such a short period of time standard bioethicists successfully claimed authority over the resolution of the issues raised by technological medicine both in the clinic and in public policy. This brings us to a second account of the origin of bioethics, which refers not to the advance of technology but to a crisis of moral authority. As an explanation of the rise of bioethics, it has two advantages. First, it addresses the loss of the moral authority of the medical profession, which was necessary for bioethics to gain moral authority, and of religious traditions, which accounts for the nature of the bioethics that gained this authority (namely, its secular and allegedly nonsectarian character). Second, it properly identifies the grounds of the claim to moral authority in bioethics, namely its confidence that it represents and articulates a common morality.

Although the history of the American bioethics movement is in its infancy there nevertheless seems to be some consensus that the movement originated when the medical profession began to turn some of its moral authority over to outsiders. This constituted a definitive break with a long tradition according to which medical ethics was the exclusive domain of the doctor (Rothman, 1990, pp. 185–187). There are various accounts of what led to this abdication of authority. Albert Jonsen argues that it began in the early 1960s in Seattle when the limited availability of a new procedure, chronic hemodialysis, "led to a radically new solution": the delegation of the task of selecting patients to a committee composed primarily of nonphysicians (Jonsen, 1993). Jonsen, a philosopher, is interested in showing how the Seattle dialysis case marked the beginning of the "new medicine" in which issues such as microallocation, which involve populations rather than individual patients, will be central to clinical practice (Jonsen, 1990). Jonsen apparently believes that most of the ethical issues raised during earlier phases of the technological transformation of medicine were in principle resolvable within the contours of an ethics internal to medicine, despite the de facto involvement of outsiders. The reason is that they were primarily questions regarding the proper treatment of individual patients. Not so the problems raised by the "new medicine," which includes genetics, disease prevention, measures of quality and futility of care, and so forth, all of which are population based rather than patient based. "Almost all the ethical problems faced by the old ethic could be resolved within the framework of a relationship between the professional and the patient; the ethical problems posed by the new medicine reflect the omnipresence of the population that stands behind that patient" (Jonsen, 1990, p. 35). The ethic internal to the medical profession has no answers for this new kind of problem.

In reality, of course, the ethic internal to medicine did not successfully resolve its problems on its own; as Jonsen acknowledges, third parties—in the form of bioethicists, patient advocates, and ultimately and most decisively, the courts—were involved early and often. From this perspective the crisis of authority derives not from the intrinsic limits of the internal ethic of medicine but from a breakdown of the confidence of outsiders in that ethic itself, those who represent it, or both. David Rothman argues that the abdication of authority began when the crisis over the ethics of human experimentation precipitated by Dr. Henry Beecher's exposure of unethical research practices brought philosophers, legislators and others into the arena of clinical research (Rothman, 1990). Rothman, a social historian, links the crisis in human experimentation to the larger rights movement of the time that curbed the discretion of constituted authorities to act in the supposed best interests of others. The linkage was assured "largely because the great majority of research subjects were minorities, drawn from the ranks of the poor, the mentally disabled, and the incarcerated" (Rothman, 1991, p. 10). Rothman concentrates on the factors that brought strangers to the bedside, but his analysis is an effort to understand how the outsider ethic, characterized by general rules or principles applied to cases, was able to replace the medical "bedside ethic," an anecdotal, case ethic taught not formally but "by example, by role modeling, by students taking cues from physicians" (Rothman, 1991, p. 9).

Despite their disagreements, therefore, Jonsen and Rothman both point to the emergence of bioethics in a crisis of moral authority that challenged either the competence or the right of the medical profession to decide all ethical issues in the practice of medicine, and that replaced an ethic internal to medicine with a very different kind of ethic. What kind of an ethic was this? When persons outside the medical profession first began to claim some authority to judge ethical issues in medical practice, they proceeded in a familiar American way: by invoking a common morality allegedly shared by everyone against a parochial morality accessible only to a priveleged few. Of course, "common morality" is an ambiguous term. It can refer to a set of universal moral beliefs or principles grounded in reason or intuition or to a philosophical reconstruction of the unsystematic, largely customary moral beliefs shared by members of a community or society. In recent years many bioethicists have shifted from the first to the second sort of account (cf. Beauchamp and Childress, 1994).

In relation to medicine the claim can take a milder form in which the author accepts what he or she takes to be the traditional moral commitments of medicine but redescribes them as a subset of the fundamental moral commitments of common morality. This was Paul Ramsey's approach (Ramsey, 1970b, pp. xi–xii). Or the claim could take a stronger form that stresses the incompatibility of traditional medical ethics with the common morality. The specter of medicine as antidemocratic and not accountable to those outside the profession was raised in the early work of Robert Veatch (Veatch, 1981, pp. 6, 89). In either case the claim is that bioethics, in distinction from traditional medical ethics, is grounded in common morality and is therefore capable of managing the new capacities of medicine.

Standard bioethics appeals to a common morality not only in contrast to a parochial professional tradition but also in the hope of overcoming the diversity and disagreement that is associated with religious traditions. In this context, the commonality is sought in secularity (or at least a limited consensus or convergence of various religious and secular beliefs), a nonsectarian posture, and standards of rationality or reasonableness that allegedly either transcend or may be shared by particular communities. However, the differences between this secular, nonsectarian, rational common morality, and religious moralities have often not been as glaring as those between the former and medical morality. One reason is that a key strategy of theologians involved in bioethical debates has been to insist that many of their moral arguments were either grounded in reason or compatible with the shared customary morality of the wider community.[6]

While few persons who accept the fact that they live in a pluralistic society would want to yield public moral authority to a particular religious tradition, the embarrassing fact remains that bioethicists do not agree on either the method or the substance of their allegedly common morality. The result, as H. Tristram Engelhardt, Jr., argues, is that standard bioethics is infected with the same irreducible diversity and endless disagreement as the religious bioethics it seeks to distinguish itself from. Moreover, this is a necessary result for any secular, nonsectarian ethics that proposes content, because moral content is impossible without particularity (Engelhardt, 1995). The tenacity with which standard bioethicists cling to their claim to articulate a common morality in spite of their disagreements testifies eloquently to the modern anxiety about moral unity in the face of diversity and to the hope that a secular rationality could supply that unity where religion failed. But if standard bioethics fails to arrive at a morality that is subtantive enough to resolve moral disagreements yet common enough to compel the rational agreement of all—if it fails, that is, to resolve the crisis of moral authority on its own grounds (i.e., rationality)—the question of why so many health professionals, bioethicists, and laypersons still find it compelling remains to be answered. My argument in what follows is that its attractiveness or worthiness has little to do with its alleged rational authority and much to do with its success in articulating and supporting certain modern moral convictions.

BIOETHICS AND THE LOSS OF TRADITION

While the second account gets the issue of moral authority right, it ignores the deeper roots of the crisis of moral authority. As a result, it fails to account for the basic moral content shared by standard bioethicists in spite of their disagreements, for the exact grounds on which traditional forms of ethics are considered inadequate, and for the kinds of issues standard bioethics fails to address due to its moral commitments. The deeper roots of the crisis of moral authority involve the loss of tradition in the West. The loss of tradition means the loss of a certain moral discourse—one that places the pursuit of health in the context of the pursuit of a good life within the limits set by fate or necessity—and its replacement by a new moral discourse—one that is dedicated to overcoming the human subjection to natural necessity. This places the narrative of the origin of bioethics squarely within a narrative of the emergence of modern moral theories.[7]

In order to describe this loss of tradition I will sketch some rather formal features of medical and religious moral traditions. The accounts are formal—I do not claim that they describe any single historically identifiable practice or community. Nor do I claim that premodern societies were marked by practices that conformed to a unified moral vision that is now lost. Rather, I offer these accounts as instances of a range of moral concerns that characterized premodern practices and communities but that modern moral discourse disavows and disallows.[8]

An adequate description of medicine as a traditional practice would clarify the relation between knowledge and technical skill, on the one hand, and health as an end for the particular patient being treated, on the other hand. As such, medicine is a practical art. It assumes an understanding of health as a standard of bodily excellence or "an activity of the living body in accordance with its excellences" (Kass, 1985, p. 174). But it also recognizes that this standard must be specified with reference to each person, so that the task is to determine the nature and degree of health appropriate for a particular patient. Hence medicine requires general knowledge about excellent bodily functioning, insight into the relation of this functioning to the capacities and roles of a particular patient, and awareness of the possibilities and limitations of facilitating or restoring functioning for this particular patient. It is impossible to achieve competence without this threefold knowledge because one can identify a skilled practitioner only by his or her ability to fulfill the possibilities and observe the limitations of bodily health for a particular patient.[9]

Three important points follow. First, the standards and ends of medicine exist in a complex relation to the practice itself: medicine is not a set of technical skills in the service of ends that can be described apart from standards of excellence of bodily functioning, but what this excellence is for any given patient involves more than the body. Second, these standards need not and will not be static. Hence there is room in principle for technological change and for growth of insight. As with any practice, "conceptions of goods and ends which the technical skills serve . . . are transformed and enriched by . . . extensions of human powers and by . . . regard for its own internal goods" (MacIntyre, 1984, p. 193). But, third, this transformation and enrichment will occur within the recognition of health as a mortal good and of human beings as destined to suffer disease and die (Kass, 1985, p. 163).

I now turn to the characteristics of the moral authority of a religious tradition. These characteristics may or may not be explicit; for some persons they may be almost entirely customary. An adequate description of such a tradition would include its account of the nature and proper ends of human beings, and of the virtues that either constitute those ends or enable one to attain them. It would also include an account of how one attains the proper ends of life, the obstacles (both internal and external) one encounters, the authorities (official or unofficial) that lead and instruct one, and the powers (for example, divine grace) that assist one. Such a tradition will also include norms, rules, and prohibitions. These specify actions or modes of conduct that are either required or ruled out in order to engage in this way of life. For example, both the major precepts of the natural law in Thomas Aquinas and the five moral precepts in Theravada Buddhism specify the necessary conditions for embarking on a way of life devoted to reaching the higher ends in each tradition. One justifies these precepts by showing how that way of life depends on observing them. Without some such norms and prohibitions it would be impossible for that way of life to be the distinctive form of belief and practice that it is. Moreover, from within such a way of life, these norms, rules, and prohibitions will have a casuistical framework in which they are refined, contested, and sometimes abandoned; conflicts between them are resolved; and rules and authorities for interpreting them are identified and contested.

Such a tradition will possess two characteristics relevant to health and illness. First, it will provide an account of how bodily health is related to the ends of life, what degree of health is necessary to attain those ends, and how suffering thwarts or helps one to realize those ends. Second, when technology brings new areas of bodily life into the realm of medical intervention, both those ends themselves and certain norms and prohibitions will place limits on the pursuit of health and the means by which it is pursued.

These characteristics of medical and religious traditions are absent in the modern moral discourse that challenged these traditions. This modern discourse, or so I argue, accounts for the cultural content on which bioethics draws. Charles Taylor's reconstruction of the sources of the modern moral self offers one fruitful way of understanding this discourse (Taylor, 1989). What follows relies heavily on key elements of Taylor's interpretation, though I alter it, add to it, and apply the resulting product to medicine. One of the chief characteristics of the modern moral discourse according to Taylor is the moral valuation of ordinary life. For Protestant Christianity human effort is fruitless in attaining salvation, which comes through divine grace alone. Hence rather than directing one's life toward the attainment of moral and religious perfection, human effort is to be directed toward serving the needs of one's neighbors. This is done by engaging in the pursuits of ordinary life such as family and work. But if the needs of one's neighbors are to be met, one's work must be disciplined and effective. It became clear beginning with Francis Bacon that effectiveness would require an instrumental approach to nature, ultimately including human nature, in order to fulfil its moral project. In this spirit Bacon praised the mechanical arts and disparaged speculative science for doing nothing "to relieve and benefit the condition of man" (Bacon, 1960, pp. 71–72; cf. Taylor, 1989, p. 213).

The instrumental approach to nature was supported by a theological conviction that God has ordered nature for the preservation and enhancement of human life. Nature is therefore governed by divine providence as in the Stoic and medieval cosmos, but the conception of a providential order has changed. The ancient and medieval conception of nature as a teleological order from which a hierarchy of ends could be derived was replaced by the burgeoning conception of nature as a law-governed mechanism, susceptible to human control and neutral with regard to ends—an order, therefore, which permits human control for the purposes of human preservation and well-being. As Taylor argues, from this perspective Baconian science could be viewed as an avenue to the fulfillment of Protestant moral and religious aspirations. Its turn from contemplation of nature to control of nature allowed nature to be used for its proper twofold purpose: to glorify God (rather than serve as an end in itself) and to benefit human beings (Taylor, 1989, pp. 231–233).[10]

Up to this point, the roots of modern morality are in Protestant Christianity. But as Taylor emphasizes, radical Enlightenment thinkers such as Jeremy Bentham were able to understand their secular agenda as a superior way of affirming ordinary life and expressing benevolence. According to them, the affirmation of ordinary life meant being true to the demands of ordinary human nature and so identifying good with pleasure and evil with pain. The Protestant commitment to meeting the needs of the neighbor now became a set of obligations to prevent and remove the causes of pain and to maximize the quantity of pleasure. As Taylor argues, this made it possible for the first time to put the relief of suffering (and the avoidance of cruelty) at the center of the social agenda. This emphasis on the relief of suffering in turn resulted in a new standard for all remaining conceptions of religious, moral, and legal order: Do they lessen the amount of suffering in the world or contribute to it? (Taylor, 1989, p. 331). From now on all these conceptions of order would have to present their credentials for relieving suffering to gain admission to the moral realm, credentials few such conceptions could produce.

Not surprisingly, this new moral agenda was closely connected with the loss of the belief in divine providence that had sustained the Protestant moral enterprise. Ever since the nominalists it had been difficult to support belief in divine providence on philosophical grounds, and as the mechanistic explanation of nature reached its climax with Newton, providential and the remaining teleological approaches to nature were both discredited. Confidence in a providential order therefore gave way to a growing emphasis on the need to extract the preservation and enhancement of human life from an indifferent nature by means of technological labor. This has implications for the approach to suffering. While the loss of ideas of providence or a meaningful cosmic order removes the incentive to find any religious or cosmic meaning for suffering, the mechanization of nature means that suffering from natural causes is no longer an inevitable feature of the world but is, to the extent that human beings are capable of controlling nature, an object of human responsibility. Hence the new worldview both requires the elimination of suffering and makes it possible.

The contrasts with traditional ways of life are clear. First, the meaning of bodily life, which was once determined by an account of its excellent functioning and limited by its subjection to fortune, will now be determined by its susceptibility to technological control. The medical wisdom of learning the limits of healing and accepting the mortality of the body will yield to Bacon's admonition to call no disease incurable and, even more presciently, to orient medical knowledge to the prolongation of life (Bacon, 1894, pp. 163, 166–168). Second, the concern with the preservation and enhancement of ordinary human nature combined with the concern to relieve suffering means that health will become an end in itself rather than a condition or a component of a virtuous life. Medical care will be devoted to relieving and eliminating suffering wherever it is found rather than to the management of health for the pursuit of virtue. Third, rules and prohibitions limiting what can be done to the body to relieve suffering will appear to be at best insufficiently concerned about suffering and at worst arbitrary and even cruelly insensitive.

This combination of technological control over nature (including the human body) and a moral commitment to relieve suffering by preventing the harms and eliminating all the conditions and limitations that threaten bodily life accounts for a large part of the nature and task of medicine in the modern era. The unquestioned commitments to technological control of the body for the sake of eliminating "misery and necessity" constitute much of what I call the Baconian project. But there is one more chapter to the story. A second aspect of the modern moral framework is what Taylor calls inwardness. Inwardness has deep Augustinian and Cartesian roots, but during the Romantic period it surfaced in the inner conviction of the importance of one's own natural fulfillment. The idea is not only that each individual is unique and original but that this uniqueness and originality determines how he or she ought to live. There is an obligation (more aesthetic than moral) for each person to live up to his or her originality (Taylor, 1989, pp. 370–376). What follows from this is the importance contemporary moderns place on free self-determination. Together with the ideal of universal benevolence, self-determination also leads to the idea of the subject as bearer of rights of immunity and entitlement. From this follows expectations that the expansion of the reign of technology over the body should be accompanied by, and in fact should make possible, the expansion of the reign of human choice over the body, and that medicine should enable and enhance whatever pattern of life one chooses.

Taylor argues that the Victorian era brought together these Enlightenment and Romanticist trends and bequeathed them to us— along with a view of history as a story of moral progress over our forebears, a progress marked by our greater sensitivity to and eradication of suffering and our greater latitude for human choice. This view enabled the Victorians to be convinced of their moral progress over the age of religion even as it enables their successors in this century to be convinced of their moral superiority over the Victorians (Taylor, 1989, pp. 393–396). As a result, medicine is based on practices and techniques of control over the body rather than on traditions of wisdom about the body. The task of public policy is to negotiate rights of immunity and entitlement rather than to determine the place of health, illness, and medical care in a well-lived and responsible life and in a good community. Traditional moral injunctions that limit or inhibit what medicine can do appear arbitrary, but there is no broader framework to evaluate and criticize the commitments of modern medicine. In the absence of such a framework the commitment to eliminate all suffering combined with an imperative to realize one's uniqueness leads to cultural expectations that medicine should eliminate whatever anyone might consider to be a burden of finitude or to provide whatever anyone might require for one's natural fulfilment. This does not mean that individual conceptions of this burden or this fulfillment are necessarily arbitrary. But it does mean that modern moral discourse provides no vocabulary with which to deliberate about what makes some such conceptions better or worse than others.

This brief sketch of modern moral discourse allows us to identify the major cultural values that standard bioethics draws on and expresses in its agenda and content. The connection of these values to the Baconian project helps explain the silence of standard bioethics on questions that challenge that project. Moreover, it shows us how this discourse, with its new ways of conceptualizing and objectifying the body and nature, and its new moral valuations, makes it impossible for the moral questions and insights of the discourse of traditional ways of life to gain a hearing. In the modern discourse, moral convictions about the place of illness and health in a morally worthy life are replaced by moral convictions about the relief of suffering and the expansion of choice, concepts of nature as ordered by a telos or governed by providence are replaced by concepts of nature as a neutral instrument that is brought into the realm of human ends by technology, and the body as object of sprirtual and moral practices is replaced by the body as object of practices of technological control. From this new perspective the moral and practical concerns of traditional discourses are obfuscated, marginalized, or rejected. But if standard bioethics derives its content and its plausibility from a contingent discourse rather than from the problems of modern technology or moral authority and its "objective" solution to these problems, a space is cleared for consideration of a bioethic that calls the agenda and content of standard bioethics, or at least their dominance or exclusivity, into question.

But before embarking on that project, three points must be made clear. First, I do not believe that there once was a golden age when medical care was grounded in a robust view of the good or that individual choices now are necessarily arbitrary. Nor do I believe that it is possible or desirable to reverse the technological revolution in medicine and simply return to traditional ways of life. Still less do I believe that publicly enforced consensus about these matters is possible or desirable. On the contrary, efforts to retrieve tradition must take account of the advantages of technology. My argument is the more modest one that modern moral discourse provides no vocabulary with which to deliberate about the meaning of corporeality, what moral purposes the body serves, what goods health should serve, or what limits the control of our bodies by technology should observe. Hence it allows for no discussion of what kinds of suffering should be eliminated, what kinds of choices human beings should make, and what role technology should play in all of this. Second, I do not argue that a commitment to the methods, theories, or principles of standard bioethics entails an explicit endorsement of the Baconian project. But neither is standard bioethics neutral with regard to that project. Negatively, the rejection of all substantive judgments about the moral meaning of bodily life and the ends technological control over the body should serve eliminates any in-principle objection to the Baconian project. Positively, standard bioethics fosters commitments to the elimination of suffering and the expansion of human choice within the moral constraints set by modern moral theories. I illustrate this positive commitment in the following chapter.

Third, my account simply identifies some features of the modern moral framework and does not do justice to the rigor with which some bioethicists have articulated and balanced these features.

Nevertheless my account allows for two conclusions in regard to the two accounts I have criticized. These conclusions should indicate why I believe my account is superior to those accounts in disclosing the moral appeal of standard bioethics. But by accomplishing this, these conclusions also indicate better than those accounts do how this moral appeal makes the quest for an alternative to standard bioethics so difficult. First, in regard to technology, it shows how the reign of technology expresses, and is perhaps in part produced by, the deepest moral commitments of modernity: the commitments to eliminate suffering and expand the range of human choices. If I am right about this, modern technology does not render traditional moralities obsolete or call for a new morality so much as it expresses and carries out an existing (modern) morality. Nor does it merely signal a will to dominate nature that levels all moral values and leads to nihilism, as many humanist and existentialist critics of technology charge.[11] Rather, modern technology is surrounded and infused by a certain kind of moral purpose. That this was the case for early prophets of technology is clear to Albert Borgmann in his summary of the projects of Francis Bacon and René Descartes.

> The main goal of these programs seems to be the domination of nature. But we must be more precise. The desire to dominate does not just spring from a lust of power, from sheer human imperialism. It is from the start connected with the aim of liberating humanity from disease, hunger, and toil, and of enriching life with learning, art, and athletics. (Borgmann, 1984, p. 36)

Indeed, one of the most characteristic features of technological medicine is the confidence among its practitioners that the elimination of suffering and the expansion of human choice, in short, the relief of human subjection to fate or necessity, are (so long as abuses in implementation are avoided) unambiguous goods whose fulfilment is made possible by technology—a confidence standard bioethics supports and defends.[12] The moral purpose that surrounds technology and the moral confidence it inspires is precisely what makes it so difficult to criticize the reign of technology in medicine—a task that would be relatively easy were modern technology simply nihilistic or were the moral purpose it represents unambiguously flawed.

Second, in regard to moral authority, the foregoing account shows why moderns allow medicine to extend its authority over new areas of life. But it offers an additional reason why standard bioethics was able to usurp much of this authority. This reason refers not to the claim of standard bioethics to articulate a common morality in place of the parochial ethic internal to medicine but to its greater success in giving individual persons a sense of control over the powers of medicine. One can divide the history of the American bioethics movement into three phases in which medical authority was challenged on these grounds. The first phase was dominated by the abuses of human experimentation documented by Beecher, and gave rise to demands for informed consent and truth telling. The second phase was dominated by the series of cases from Karen Ann Quinlan to Nancy Beth Cruzan that established the right of patients to the termination of life-sustaining treatment. This phase continues in the current controversies over physician-assisted death. The third phase may have begun with the Helga Wanglie case and will decide whether or not patients (or their surrogates) can demand medical treatment that their physicians believe is medically ineffective. Each phase can be interpreted in terms of a struggle in which medical authority defined by the ethic internal to medicine was (or will be) subordinated to the authority of the choice of the individual patient. Once again, the challenge to standard bioethics faces a greater challenge from this perspective. The claim of standard bioethics to have articulated a common morality is open to immediate objections. Engelhardt's argument that there is not only disagreement among the theories themselves but that any moral content assumes particularity is relevant here. The argument that standard bioethics is not really neutral toward all views of the good but rather articulates its own thin view of the good whose main features are roughly those I have described in this section is a hard-won argument, but has clear evidence in its favor. However, it is not immediately clear, and thus is much more difficult to show (as I try to show in my discussion of Foucault in chapter seven), that standard bioethics has actually failed to give authority and control over technology to individuals rather than to medicine (or to society through medicine), or that gaining such control for its own sake is not the ultimate purpose of bioethics.

It is one thing, therefore, to challenge the self-understanding of standard bioethics by pointing out the moral discourse that lends it its agenda, content, and plausibility; it is quite another (and much more difficult) thing to argue that its moral purpose and its understanding of human freedom are inadequate and to argue for an alternative agenda and content for bioethics. Fortunately, as the following chapters indicate, arguments for such an alternative are as old as the bioethics movement itself. Unfortunately, as I will argue in several of these chapters, many of these arguments concede too much to the modern moral framework to supply an alternative to it.

CONCLUSION

What, then, is the origin of the agenda of standard bioethics? The discourse in which religious and medical traditions were displaced. And what gives this agenda its plausibility? Its support of the effort to control natural necessity in the absence of the capacity to find any moral or spiritual place for the body as finite, mortal, and subject to fortune. To question standard bioethics, therefore, is to question the most fundamental assumption of a society rooted in the Baconian project: the assumption that in the absence of such a capacity, the power of technology over our lives has truly benefited us and has truly made us more self-determining. Whether these values and this assumption will survive new crises such as micro- and macroallocation and the appropriateness of genetic interventions, or whether these crises will lead to a recognition of the limits to and the costs of the effort to relieve the human condition is unknown. What is clear is that these limits and these costs have been the subject matter of a countermovement in bioethics whose major figures I examine in the chapters that follow. But before turning to the countermovement, it is necessary to say more about how standard bioethics supports the Baconian project. To that task I now turn.

CHAPTER 2

Standard Bioethics
and the Baconian Project

This chapter examines arguments about physician-assisted death and germ-line gene therapy in order to exhibit the characteristics and limitations of standard bioethics mentioned in chapter 1. Some readers may question why I have chosen these two issues. After all, it seems unlikely that either of them will ever be applied to large numbers of people. Nevertheless these two issues exemplify the more general effort of technological medicine to relieve the human condition by expanding choice and eliminating suffering. I trust that the ensuing discussion will make their exemplary status more clear.

PHYSICIAN-ASSISTED DEATH

Standard bioethicists appear to be slowly building a consensus according to which the primary morally significant characteristic of physician-assisted suicide and euthanasia is the presence or absence of self-determination on the part of the patient.[1] In other words, if the conditions for self-determination are met (decision-making capacity, absence of depression or temporary rage or frustration, etc.) and the physician consents, then an act of physician-assisted death is presumably justified. Most arguments of this sort also make room for procedural safeguards and other restrictions. But the justificatory work done by the value of self-determination is central if not exclusive, at least where single acts of physician-assisted death are concerned. Now that self-determination is generally enshrined as the sole or primary morally relevant feature of individual acts of physician-assisted death, the question has shifted to whether consequences of its practice should prevent physician-assisted death, justifiable though particular cases of it may be, from being morally acceptable as a practice or a policy.

I have referred to a consensus, but of course there are some who interpret the progression from the right to reject useless and unwanted medical treatment to the moral permissibility of acts of physician-assisted killing—a progression whose curve very nearly defines the past twenty years of bioethics—as a slide down a slippery slope. According to this narrative of moral decline, the growing acceptability of physician-assisted death indicates the abandonment of an uncompromising commitment to human life that medicine and indeed western society allegedly stand for. I suspect, however, that most secular bioethicists would endorse K. Danner Clouser's narrative of moral progress. Clouser views this same progression "as a gradual recognition, the gradual discovery, of one's right of self-determination over against tradition, law, and technology. At each stage, the traditional emotions attaching to that action had to be overcome in the course of reasserting self-determination, and so on to the next stage" (Clouser, 1991, p. 307).

I do not intend to moderate this conflict of interpretations. What interests me is that each narrative understands the process itself as a series of efforts to draw morally significant lines between an acceptable activity and killing. Clouser identifies the various points at which lines were drawn and redrawn: At first withdrawing any treatment was considered killing while withholding treatment was "allowing to die." Gradually withdrawing "extraordinary" but not "ordinary" treatment became a form of letting die. Finally, withdrawing certain kinds of "ordinary" treatment (e.g., nutrition and hydration) eventually came to be seen as a way of "helping" patients die rather than killing them (Clouser, 1991, p. 307). Clouser oversimplifies a very complex process, but the point is clear: at each stage a line was drawn between killing the patient and letting or helping him or her die of the underlying disease process. Until recently, then, advocacy of self-determination in physician-assisted death has had to overcome resistance on the grounds that the latter, in distinction from withholding or withdrawing treatment, constitutes killing the patient rather than letting him or her die or letting the disease kill him or her. Among standard bioethicists, Daniel Callahan and Susan Wolf have attempted to oppose one or another form of physician-assisted death by distinguishing killing from letting die (Callahan, 1989; Wolf, 1989). I am not competent to judge Wolf's claim that the legal permissibility of refusal and abatement of treatment has depended on the continuing legal prohibition of euthanasia, so that acceptance of the latter would jeopardize the legal status of the former.

However, it seems clear that the view that stopping life support could be distinguished from killing in the eyes of many persons was a major factor in the acceptance of the moral permissibility of the former. By the same token, if the distinction between killing and allowing to die were found to be irrelevant in at least some acts of stopping life support, then their permissibility might be able to be extended to acts of physician-assisted death. In other words, the line between withholding and withdrawing treatment, on the one hand, and physician-assisted death, on the other hand, depends to a large extent on the claim that the second but not the first involves intentional killing. If this claim is untrue, then insofar as the distinction depends on it, either both sets of acts are impermissible or neither is.

There is no need to repeat here the well-known arguments against certain formulations of the distinctions between withholding and withdrawing life-sustaining treatment or between killing and letting die. I will only repeat those of their conclusions that have gained wide acceptance and that relate to the issue I am considering. First, the distinction between withholding and withdrawing treatment is conceptually unclear in some cases and the distinction between act and omission that underlies it is unclear in such cases and morally irrelevant in other cases (cf. Beauchamp and Childress, 1994, pp. 196–200). Second, the distinction between killing and letting die rests in many cases on a mistaken view of causality. In Dan Brock's example, the morally relevant distinction between the act of a physician who removes a respirator from a patient at her request and the act of her greedy son who removes it in order to claim his inheritance is not whether the disease killed the person (in both cases the act of removing the respirator killed the person) or whether death is intended (in both cases it is), but in other features of the two acts: the motives of each agent, the consent of the patient, the social sanction for the act of the physician (Brock, 1992, p. 13; cf. Beauchamp and Childress, 1994, pp. 219–225). One who accepts this line of argument need not believe that these distinctions are always irrelevant and may continue to affirm that in some cases death is not intended simply by removing a respirator from a patient—cases, for example, when the patient would die in roughly the same amount of time whether artificially ventilated or not. But in many and perhaps most cases, the morally relevant issue would be whether or not the killing is justified, not whether the act is an act of killing or letting die. And if one believes that removal of a respirator by a physician from a consenting patient whose death would otherwise have been delayed can be justified, then there seems to be no reason why other forms of intentional killing under similar conditions and in similar circumstances cannot be justified.

For purposes of this chapter I will not develop my hunch that a more adequate understanding of intentions or recognition of other morally relevant features may distinguish at least some acts of abatement of treatment from suicide and euthanasia.[2] My point is only that with the growing recognition among standard bioethicists that stopping life support constitutes intentional killing, their efforts to draw a line between these acts and acts of physician-assisted death have failed. This resolves the strictly moral issue in favor of permitting physician-assisted death and leaves two nonmoral issues, one prudential and one consequential, unresolved. The prudential issue concerns questions about whether and when patients are making a self-determining choice and who is capable of judging it. Should those who make such requests be presumed to be clinically depressed? Should psychiatric evaluations be conducted before the physician assists in a patient's death? Should the patient be required to repeat a request for assistance in dying on multiple occasions over a certain period of time? These questions indicate that procedural safeguards may be needed to guarantee to the extent possible that requests are genuinely self-determining.

These prudential questions already merge into the issue of consequences. Even if individual acts of physician-assisted suicide are justifiable, would physician-assisted death as an accepted practice or policy lead to ill consequences that could override its justifiability? Three sets of questions are especially relevant. The first, which relates to the prudential issues surrounding self-determination, is whether the general acceptability of physician-assisted death would encourage its extension to those who do not want or request it. Will pressure from burdened families or institutions coerce some to request it even though they do not desire it? Will societal protection of those whose quality of life is judged too low or whose cost to society is judged too high erode if physician-assisted death is a live option for them? The second set of questions asks whether the societal commitment to providing optimal care for the dying or devoting resources to the development of new forms of pain relief will erode if dying patients can simply opt for suicide or euthanasia. The third set of questions asks whether the trust of the public in the medical profession or the trust of individual patients in their physicians will erode if doctors are perceived as those who assist in death.

These consequential considerations deserve a lengthy discussion, but for my purposes it is enough to note two points. First, as with all consequentialist arguments immediate and certain consequences take priority over remote and uncertain consequences. Second, self-determination and relief of suffering rank high in the value system of standard bioethics as well as being both immediate and certain, while the consequences mentioned above are all uncertain and somewhat remote. Moreover, as Brock argues, the very grounds on which physician-assisted death is permitted—that is, self-determination—should itself prevent at least the first set of ill consequences (extension to those who do not want or request it) from occurring given appropriate procedural safeguards (Brock, 1992, pp. 20f.). It seems quite clear, then, that for most standard bioethicists there are no serious moral hindrances to the permissibility of physician-assisted death. Recognition of self-determination combined with procedural safeguards (such as full information, repeated requests, and consideration of all alternatives) and other restrictions (such as requiring that the patient be in a terminal condition) to reduce the likelihood of the most serious consequences seems to cover what is morally at stake in the issue of physician-assisted death.

From this brief survey, the evolution of the treatment of physician-assisted death seems to conform perfectly to the first two models of the origins of bioethics considered in chapter one. Life-extending technology seems to have rendered a traditional norm—the prohibition of intentional killing—inapplicable by showing how it entangles us in distinctions that technological medicine has gradually found to be obsolete. Moreover, it is not clear why we should have attached so much importance to intentional killing in the first place; by the time standard bioethics had erased the lines drawn against it, it was difficult to understand why so much ink had been used up drawing the line. This seems to support the idea that standard bioethics had replaced a tradition that had lost its authority with a universal moral principle, self-determination.

Of course, it is not surprising that standard bioethics would represent this evolutionary process in these terms; as I noted in chapter one, such terms are favorable to its cause. I will not discuss whether traditions are able to continue to distinguish various forms of abating treatment from intentional killing or whether most standard bioethicists treat self-determination as a good rather than a side constraint and thus claim common moral authority for what is in reality yet another particular conception of the proper ends of medicine, though I think the answer to all of these questions is a resounding yes. Instead I want to show how standard bioethics, by constructing the issue of physician-assisted death in these terms, fails to understand physician-assisted death as part of a larger effort to control death. As a result, standard bioethics is unable to understand how this effort shapes our practices of dying and extends the control of medicine over our lives. In order to make this clear, I will show how physician-assisted death is viewed from the perspective of my third model of the origins of bioethics, and will point out two moral concerns that follow.

The third model views the evolution of attitudes toward physician-assisted death in light of a complex relation between medicine and our quest for control over fate. Traditionally, medicine by necessity either withdrew in the face of death or changed its strategy from curing to caring. In both cases medicine recognized death as its limit. Attitudes toward death itself and practices surrounding dying—ranging from where it usually occurred to how the dying person and his or her survivors understood their responsibilities toward one another—reflected this powerlessness of medicine. In contrast to this, a primary task of medicine in the modern era, as Bacon foresaw, has been to extend our lives indefinitely. This task was welcomed because most people were convinced that it would bring into the sphere of choice what had once belonged to fate, namely our dying. But of course, the power of medicine itself soon became its own form of fate as the capacity to keep people alive far outpaced their capacity to maintain control over their lives. The very reason for gaining control over death was in danger of being lost. Given this situation, if medicine were to succeed in its appointed role of delivering us from fate, it would have to find a way to restore control over dying to self-determining choice. Hence physician-assisted death. In short, the evolution toward the permissibility of physician-assisted death embodies two assumptions: that we should be able to control death, and that it is the task of medicine to give us this control.

Because standard bioethics is committed to both assumptions, it is unable to recognize two problems connected with them. The first involves the power of medicine over our lives. From this vantage point we can understand why the control we have sought has been so elusive—namely because we can expand our self-determination only by giving medicine more power. There is, in effect, a sort of antinomy of freedom involved in the effort to control death: self-determination comes through technological control, which in turn means the control of medicine over our lives. Thus our dying is subjected to the full range of medical control: technological devices, bureacratic monitoring, and the pressures on both patients and caregivers to subject dying to rationalized decision-making procedures and imperatives of expediency. That physician-assisted death could free us from the devices is possible (though not certain); that it will entangle us further in the other phenomena is inevitable.

The second problem is that the effort to control death governs contemporary practices of dying just as thoroughly as the traditional withdrawal in the face of death governed past practices. In its effort to bring dying into the sphere of choice, standard bioethics ignores questions of what conditions drive persons to choose an early death, what destroys the capacity of seriously ill persons to affirm their lives as worthwhile, what responsibilities those who are dying and those whom they will leave behind have toward one another, and so on. Standard bioethics is unable to question contemporary practices of dying along these lines because it is concerned only with ensuring that such practices allow for self-determination. But self-determination is vacuous if the societal and medical practices that govern the dying process make senses of abandonment and worthlessness an almost inevitable part of dying, for many substantive choices require a community of care and a sense of worth.

By now my point should be clear. Standard bioethics participates in the Baconian project and is unable to raise moral questions concerning that project. Moreover, its representation of the issue of physician-assisted death as the shifting and erasure of a line between justifiable expressions of self-determination and intentional killing obscures its own support of the Baconian project. The result is that standard bioethics leaves us unaware of how our moral identities are determined by the ambitions of Baconian medicine and unable to resist this determination and enlist technology in the service of a responsible and well-lived life. It should be clear from this that I am not interested in arguing for a prohibition against physician-assisted death any more than I am arguing for the sufficiency of self-determination. To cast the issue in these terms is to perpetuate the very moral discourse I am calling into question. And I am not arguing for a return to pretechnological ways of dying—on the contrary, one of my major points is that our moral projects must both resist technological control and enlist technology in their service. This points to a complex relation to technology rather than an outright rejection of it. In short, our desire to control fate and expand choice will continue to entangle us in these pervasive and subtle forms of medical control unless this desire is transformed by our moral projects. Moreover, unless our practices of dying embody our moral projects, our capacity to die in accordance with our projects— that is, to die as we genuinely choose—will, ironically, be undermined by the contemporary practices we have set up to ensure that death will be brought under the dominion of choice.

Standard bioethicists will likely respond by arguing that no such moral project can be made universally binding and that the success of standard bioethics in establishing self-determination makes it possible for all such projects to flourish. The first point is certainly true, but the second point is dubious. For, as we have seen, standard bioethics does not simply argue for self-determination as a necessary side constraint that disavows all moral content. Rather, it represents itself as rendering a traditional norm obsolete, and it participates in an ongoing effort to gain control over death. Hence the self-determination it promises is inadequate at best, illusory at worst. The capacity to live out a moral project of one's choosing, and to be supported by others in it, is necessary if the powers of medicine to extend and end life are to serve human purposes rather than determine them, frustrate them, or manage them.

HUMAN GERM-LINE GENE THERAPY

A bioethical issue that has evoked similar efforts to draw lines between morally acceptable and unacceptable interventions is human germ-line gene therapy. From the time scientists began to come to terms with the possibilities of recombinant DNA (rDNA) research, germ-line therapy has evoked sustained controversy. After developments in molecular genetics prompted a brief self-imposed moratorium on rDNA research, the National Institutes of Health issued guidelines for continuing such research in 1976. In 1982 the President's Commission for the Study of Ethical Problems in Medicine and Biomedical and Behaviorial Research, which met from 1976 to 1983, produced a report recommending that research on somatic cell therapy be carried out under approval of an oversight committee but that research on human germ-line cells not be carried out. Until the early 1990s the line between research into human somatic cell therapy and research into human germ-line therapy was widely accepted as the line between what is morally permissible and what is not (Fletcher, 1990).

In retrospect it is clear both why it seemed appropriate to many to draw a line here and why such a line was bound to be unstable given the state of research and the preoccupations of standard bioethics. First, during the 1980s somatic cell therapy in the form of transfer of a normally functioning gene into host cells became progressively more technically feasible while similar progress was not being made in the feasibility of germ-line therapy (Anderson, 1989). But this involved a lag that was not likely to last forever. Although the results of gene transfer and replacement in nonhuman preimplantation embryos have been mixed, it is a reasonable assumption that they will continue to improve. Second, while somatic cell therapy is carried out with the consent of the patient, germ-line gene therapy has potentially enormous effects on future generations of persons who would be modified according to our lights and without their consent. Moreover, assuming, as is most likely, that it would be carried out on embryos rather than adults, it would involve experimentation on subjects who are unable to give their consent. But, as I will discuss in the following chapter in connection with Hans Jonas, it has been notoriously difficult to justify ascriptions of rights to future persons on purely philosophical grounds. It has been similarly difficult to secure such rights for embryos on these grounds. Third, germ-line therapy greatly expands the range of consequences of our interventions and thus the risks they involve. Given our vast ignorance about the human genome, we may eliminate deleterious genes that, unknown to us, are essential to human survival of an unforeseeable future threat. However, this risk would apply equally to widespread use of somatic cell therapy and of other rDNA technology (Munson and Davis, 1992, pp. 147–148). Moreover, any such threat is highly uncertain while the benefits of eliminating serious diseases from the germ line would be immediate and obvious. Fourth, germ-line interventions bring into the realm of feasibility the worst eugenic scenarios. It seems impossible to forestall a mad rush to design our descendents according to our ideals and to avoid the gross inequalities and discrimination that would likely follow. But since it is not clear in the first place to what extent various capacities are genetically determined, it is difficult to determine how much of a threat this is. Furthermore, concerns about eugenics per se and about the resulting inequality and discrimination would apply also to somatic cell therapy; germ-line alterations introduce problems of scale but not of kind. Similar arguments also apply to a fifth point, that germ-line interventions involve "playing God" in a way that somatic cell interventions or all the other ways in which human actions and decisions have determined their descendents do not. Again, it is a question of the efficacy of genetic factors alone and a matter of degree rather than of kind.

I do not wish to evaluate these arguments, but only to point out that they seem to have led to a rough consensus that the line between somatic cell and germ-line interventions is in most cases morally insignificant. This is not to say that those who agree with some version of these arguments endorse research into and implementation of germ-line therapy whenever it becomes technically feasible. For it may always result in relatively low rates of success and relatively high risks, and it may never be cost-effective. My point is that all these considerations involve distinctions of degree between somatic cell interventions and germ-line interventions rather than distinctions of principle.

During much of the time the line between somatic cell and germ line was being drawn and then questioned in the ways I have just sketched, W. French Anderson and John C. Fletcher, both individually and in collaboration, have advocated research into germ-line therapy and have argued for drawing a line not between somatic cell therapy and germ-line therapy, where it was traditionally drawn, but between both of these, on the one hand, and enhancement of human characteristics not directly implicated in disease, on the other hand. In a joint article Fletcher and Anderson note that a new stage of the debate is dawning, one that will distinguish between therapy and enhancement rather than somatic cell and germ line (Fletcher and Anderson, 1992). They propose a five-point agenda for the debates that will constitute this new level. The first point is a purely scientific matter. It concerns the degree of conclusiveness of research with transgenic animals for human embryos. As I have noted, this research is promising but inconclusive; gene transfer into nonhuman preimplantation embryos has a low rate of success and can not yet be made site-specific. The second point is largely moral: What should be the ethical and scientific criteria for determining when it is ethical to begin learning about the feasibility and safety of germ-line interventions in human embryos? The third point concerns the priority of germ-line research relative to other types of research. The fourth point considers whether clear moral lines can be drawn to prevent abuses. The fifth point consists of a list of broader issues: whether there is a moral obligation to future generations to prevent genetic disorders, whether genetic diagnosis and therapy can be distributed equitably, whether germ-line therapy will invest a too-radical power in the hands of a few, whether it will harmfully alter cultural conceptions of being human, whether the experiments will violate human dignity, and whether germ-line therapy will "transgress limits of permissible human powers and, theologically viewed, assume powers that ought to be attributed only to a Creator" (Fletcher and Anderson, 1992, pp. 28–29).

Fletcher and Anderson quite prudently announce that they will discuss only the first three of these points. But the question is whether the framework of standard bioethics they employ in their analysis allows them to say anything at all about many of the matters raised by points four and five. The key to Fletcher and Anderson's argument is in their response to point two on the criteria for learning about germ-line interventions in embryos. Following an application of the standard principles of bioethics to this question they turn to the proper goals of biomedical research: "Goals for biomedical research should be set primarily to cure and prevent the greatest sources of human suffering and premature death, and to relieve the pain and suffering caused by these disorders." They then argue that the principles of beneficence and nonmaleficence "create imperatives to relieve and prevent basic causes of human suffering. It follows from this ethical imperative that society ought not to draw a moral line between intentional germ-line therapy and somatic cell therapy." Instead the line should be drawn between both of these and enhancement by either mode of therapy (Fletcher and Anderson, 1992, pp. 30–31). In other words, obligations to prevent and remove evil derived from the principles of nonmaleficence and beneficence render in-principle objections to germ-line therapy immoral, though of course other factors such as safety, cost-effectiveness, and relative priority may justifiably determine whether research or implementation are in fact carried out. But the same obligations do not extend this justifiability to the use of either somatic cell or germ-line interventions for the enhancement of various human traits, since these by definition do not involve "basic causes of human suffering." Moreover, since (as we will see) enhancement violates other moral principles we are justified in drawing a line against this use of genetic technology in both its somatic cell and germ-line forms.

However, the effort to draw a line between therapy and enhancement is frought with difficulties. Sheldon Krimsky has pointed out that the line between somatic cells and germ cells is scientifically clear since the cells are distinct biological entities and it is possible to make measurements that distinguish between alterations of these cells. By contrast, the line between amelioration of disease and enhancement of traits has no such scientific basis. Moreover, any trait that has a significant association with the onset of a disease can be thought of as a proto-disease and thus as a candidate for genetic intervention on Fletcher and Anderson's own grounds (Krimsky, 1990, pp. 172–173). Indeed, following up on this last point, one could imagine numerous traits whose enhancement by gene therapy would make one less susceptible to a disease. In response to these points, Fletcher and Anderson simply repeat Charles Culver and Bernard Gert's category of "malady" to distinguish what conditions involve suffering from disease and which involve characteristics unrelated to disease. But the category itself is inadequate to do the work Fletcher and Anderson require of it: since medicine already treats conditions other than what Culver and Gert recognize as maladies the category is too formal to resolve controversies about what counts as a malady, and it does not tell us what to do with traits that contribute to or are associated with maladies.

The point, however, is not only that the line between therapy and enhancement itself is fuzzy or that there are conditions that call such a line into question. This is true enough, but there are two more basic points. The first is that the principles of beneficence and nonmaleficence alone cannot generate meaningful distinctions between different types of suffering without a broader account of the role of health, illness, and medical care in our lives and communities. This is especially the case in a modern moral framework where there is a strong emphasis on individual choice so that in principle each individual decides what for him- or herself constitutes suffering and its relief. Fletcher and Anderson try to substitute a purely formal or technical definition of suffering where only a normative account will do. The second point is that even if a distinction between suffering due to a malady and suffering from the human condition could be made Fletcher and Anderson have given no convincing reasons for drawing a line there. They argue that enhancement would violate the ethical norms that currently govern negative eugenics and that the devotion of scarce resources to enhancement would violate principles of distributive justice. But given the unresolved controversies about distributive justice and the confidence of most standard bioethicists in the safeguards against what they consider the worst abuses of positive eugenics (i.e., those that violate the self-determining choices of individuals), these reasons are unlikely to bear the weight Fletcher and Anderson place on them.[3]

In short, to draw a line between therapy and enhancement requires a much richer account of suffering than Fletcher and Anderson can provide using the principles of standard bioethics. It is therefore not surprising that standard bioethicists are increasingly rejecting efforts to draw a line here (cf. Resnik, 1994). Viewed in this light, the inability of Fletcher and Anderson to address their own points about power, conceptions of the human, permissible limits, and so forth loom large. For it is insight on issues such as these that is needed to develop the larger normative framework that can make distinctions between what counts as genuine suffering or an undesirable trait and what does not. Standard bioethics, in other words, does not allow them to mark out and defend the very moral distinction that is central to their own proposal. Moreover, standard bioethics prevents them from reflecting on the moral discourse in which relief of suffering actually inheres and thus from understanding why their proposal is necessarily unstable—namely because standard bioethics is forced to define as suffering to be relieved by medicine whatever anyone considers to be suffering. Finally, it leaves them no way of resisting the power of genetic medicine to determine our wants and thus bring us under its control. For example, it is significant that neither Fletcher and Anderson nor other standard bioethicists pay attention to the immense social pressures on persons to make the "right" genetic decisions for their descendents, or to the relentless monitoring that will be required over generations to determine the efficacy of germ-line therapy. In short, standard bioethics offers Fletcher and Anderson no perspective from which to discuss some of the most profound implications of germ-line interventions. Far less does it tell us how these new powers can serve our moral projects without determining them.

I have chosen Fletcher and Anderson precisely because, unlike many standard bioethicists, they are concerned enough about these deeper issues to note their importance. My problem with them is not that I disagree with their conclusion regarding therapy and enhancement, but that, as is becoming increasingly clear, the distinction is illusory without a moral framework that can qualify the relief of suffering and make it possible to determine what kind and degree of power medicine will have over our lives. But the discourse of standard bioethics makes it impossible even to discuss what kind of a moral framework would accomplish this.

CONCLUSION

Much could be said about the penchant of bioethics for drawing and then erasing lines. From a social-psychological perspective it doubtless reflects a collective anxiety about the powers technology has unleashed and the loss, for many, of religious or moral traditions that can give authoritative or convincing answers regarding the use of these powers. From a broader cultural perspective, it may exhibit what Albert Jonsen has described as a process in which bioethics has gradually overcome American moralism (Jonsen, 1991). But the perspective I have sketched suggests another interpretation, namely that standard bioethics has succeeded in bringing its moral commitments to bear against the remnants of previous kinds of moral discourse. According to its self-understanding, standard bioethics has provided solutions to the moral dilemmas raised by technology by articulating common principles. But in fact standard bioethics has inscribed us deeper into the Baconian project. It has provided the moral grounds for the effort to relieve the human condition of subjection to death and to a genetic fate. But because it is incapable of determining what practices of dying best serve our moral projects and what kinds of suffering interfere with those projects, it cannot tell us what kinds of suffering to relieve or what choices to make. As a result it leaves us at the mercy of the power of medicine (or of society through medicine) to control us, determine our "preferences," and subject our dying and our provisions for our descendents to its ruthless demands of expediency.

An analysis of the approaches of standard bioethics to physician-assisted death and germ-line gene therapy does not constitute a decisive argument against standard bioethics. Far less does it constitute an argument for an alternative. But I believe it is illustrative of the shortcomings of standard bioethics. As for an alternative, several will be considered in the following chapters as I now begin the task of exploring those who have criticized the Baconian project and rejected many of the assumptions of standard bioethics.

CHAPTER 3

Utopia, Nihilism,
and the Quest for Responsibility

In a brief intellectual autobiography Hans Jonas describes how in the late 1960s "the emergence of the most acute, internal crisis of the Baconian ideal" woke him from his complacency about the perils of technology and set the scholarly task that would govern the last quarter century of his distinguished career (Jonas, 1974, p. xvi). What shattered this complacency was the ecological crisis and developments in human (especially genetic) engineering—in other words, the growing threat to the biosphere that sustains human life and the capacity to refashion human life through genetic, biochemical, and neurological interventions. The latter concern, Jonas argues, calls for a normative conception or image of the human in order to determine proper uses and moral limits of our refashioning capacities. The following two chapters examine, respectively, the efforts by Jonas and James Gustafson to arrive at such a normative conception of the human. Their efforts differ on many points, as will become clear. But they are united on at least four points. First, the powers of technology that render the question of the normatively human so acute and urgent are imbedded in a broader scientific and techno-logical framework that renders traditional conceptions of the norma-tively human inadequate. Second, an adequate conception of the human follows largely from a proper understanding of the place of human beings in nature—in contrast to the misunderstanding of humanity and nature that fuels the Baconian project. This in turn raises questions about the modern subject and his presumptions of control over a world he bends to his purposes. Third, this approach will not be able to deliver either the certainty or the robust content that was traditionally claimed for normative conceptions of the human. Fourth, medicine, especially biomedical research, is a primary arena in which the internal crisis of the Baconian project emerges, and in which the failure to arrive at a normative conception of the human would be most devastating.

TECHNOLOGY AND THE DIALECTICS OF POWER

For Jonas, technology is "the focal fact of modern life," in the sense that it "touches on almost everything vital to man's existence" (Jonas, 1979, p. 34). He shares this pervasive understanding of technology with others who view it as more than merely an instrument for human purposes, notably Martin Heidegger.[1] But what distinguishes Jonas is a dialectical view of technology that is never made explicit in his writings but nevertheless governs his project. The dialectic is a dialectic of power, specifically the power of the modern subject. Simply put, the very technology that originates in the effort of the modern subject to bring the external world under his power ends with the power of technology to recoil back and destroy or radically refashion the very subject whose power it is. The chief question for Jonas is how to gain power over this power without succumbing to the dialectic. Since the dialectic is inseparable from the modern subject, his answer lies in an ethic that partially (though not fully, as we will see) breaks with the modern subject. It accomplishes the break by showing how what comes under my power is committed to my care inasmuch as it is an objective good that confronts my power with its intrinsic right to be. The task for this post-Baconian ethic is therefore to arrive at a conception of the human as an objective good that we are responsible for maintaining against the threats posed to it by our technological power.

This chapter describes the dialectic of power that characterizes the modern subject and is played out through a peculiar combination of nihilism and utopianism, and reconstructs Jonas's alternative to it. But in order to understand why Jonas believes his alternative is necessary, one must first understand the challenges modern technology poses to any ethic.

THE PREDICAMENT OF ETHICS

The nature of modern technology and its place in modern life challenge the most basic assumptions of traditional ethical thought, assumptions that persist in modern ethics, including standard bioethics.

Jonas argues that forms of ethics in antiquity shared three tacit and interconnected premises: that the human condition is given in the nature of things, that the human good is determinable on that basis, and that the range of human action and responsibility are narrowly circumscribed (Jonas, 1984, p. 1). The problem is that modern technology has rendered all three of these premises obsolete, but modern moral theories (including standard bioethics) proceed as if they were still operative. The first premise presupposes that human action cannot harm or radically alter nature (including human nature), whose order is immutable and thus invulnerable to human intrusions into it (Jonas, 1984, p. 3). The principles and concepts of previous forms of ethics therefore dealt exclusively with the sociopolitical realm, where the order of things could be affected by human actions. This immunity of nature clearly no longer holds. Human causal power now extends the domain of responsibility to objects, including the biosphere itself, that once provided the unalterable backdrop for all human moral concerns. The existence of human beings on earth, once a given, is now an object of obligation for which a rational justification must be given (Jonas, 1984, p. 10). Potential capacities for radical expansion of the life span, control of behavior, and manipulation of the genome raise questions about what is normatively human while putting human nature itself at stake (Jonas, 1984, pp. 18–21).

The second premise of premodern ethics presupposes that knowledge of the nature of things also yields knowledge of the human good. This had implications for the nature and status of various kinds of knowing. The impossibility of altering nature assured that *techne* would remain ethically neutral insofar as its interventions into nature had no power to fundamentally alter or destroy nature, but also inferior insofar as it confronted nature as a realm of necessity which it was powerless to overcome. As such, *techne* was "a measured tribute to necessity, not the road to mankind's chosen goal" (Jonas, 1984, p. 9). That goal involved contemplation or *theoria*, which, far from being ethically neutral, had for its object the highest good. To act against the good was therefore to act in contradiction to knowledge. Bacon was the first to articulate the stunning reversal of this hierarchy of *theoria* and *techne*. The chosen goal of human beings is no longer contemplation of things but power over them. Jonas draws out the implications of the reversal. "At its most modest, it means elevating *homo faber* to the essential aspect of man. At its most extravagant, it means elevating power to the position of his dominant and interminable goal" (Jonas, 1979, p. 38). As *techne*, knowledge can supply neither the motivation nor the standard for its own power over nature. The motivation must come from the charity or benevolence that motivates the knower to use *techne* to fulfill human need and eliminate misery. But charity or benevolence supplies no standard for its use, which can only come from a conception of the good (Jonas, 1966, pp. 194–197). In short, whereas *techne*, because it is no longer innocent in its effects, loses its ethical neutrality, knowledge, because it is reduced to *techne*, loses its capacity to know the good. Knowledge can therefore be used without inconsistency for good or evil, and experts will not necessarily have the capacity to determine proper and improper uses of their knowledge.[2]

The third premise of premodern ethics presupposes that the effects of human action are of limited expanse and duration. In the premodern world, actions and their consequences transpired in the temporal present and in the presence of the recipient of the action. There was therefore no need for either long-range responsibility or long-range predictive knowledge. Even where premodern forms of ethics were future-oriented, as in their concern with an afterlife or the future life of the state or community, they assumed that what is required for the afterlife or for the duration of the state or community is what is morally right or good in the present and at all times (Jonas, 1984, pp. 12–15). In contrast, human actions now set causal chains in motion that have profound effects on spatially and temporally distant objects and peoples. Apart from their magnitude, the irreversibility of many of these actions ensures that corrections of errors will be more difficult and the freedom to make them more restricted, while their cumulativity ensures that actions that occur later in a temporal process will not occur under the same conditions as the initial actions but will build on previous conditions. These linear features keep technology constantly on the verge of catastrophe while also rendering the lessons of experience, with their cyclical assumptions, inapplicable (Jonas, 1984, pp. 7, 31–32).

If Jonas's description is correct, modern technology has radically undermined the entire framework of human action that standard bioethics assumes in its principles and concepts.[3] If bioethics were to address seriously the nature and scope of human action in the technological era, it would have to address the moral significance of human nature itself, to determine whether there are any objective goods at which *techne* aims, and to evaluate morally the effects of our actions on a future we determine but cannot predict or control. But one of Jonas's most persistent points is that the very technology that issues this challenge to ethics also destroys the very grounds for developing any such ethic. This predicament of ethics becomes clear when we understand modern technology in its relation to the modern view of reality and its ethos.

NIHILISTIC UTOPIANISM

Current theories of modernity often find the key to modernity in the Cartesian *cogito* and the epistemology or form of subjectivity that followed from it. For Jonas also Descartes is a certain watershed, but for different reasons. While Bacon conceived the modern subject who would subdue the earth for his benevolent purposes, Jonas argues that Descartes articulated the world in which this subject and his project could flourish. Descartes marks the point at which western dualism reached its greatest articulation, and realized the subject as the sole center of purpose and value set over against all that is external and available for his use. Of course, under the pressure of his rigorous formulation, dualism itself collapsed into a competition between materialism and the philosophy of consciousness—a competition that confirmed the banishment of value and purpose from nature and into the will which dualism had begun.

When Descartes succeeded in describing nature as pure extension, he completed the shattering of the ancient notion of kinship between humanity and nature that Judaism and Christianity had begun and Gnosticism had accomplished in its own way.[4] This left human beings to inhabit a nature devoid of its own purposes and indifferent to human purposes (Jonas, 1966, pp. 70–72, 213–214). The key to this process was the success of early modern physics in explaining the movements of heavenly bodies by the same laws of mechanics applicable to earthly bodies. While the substantial forms that constituted the ancient cosmos had assured, in their rational order, both a kinship with the human logos and a hierarchical order, the scientific revolution reduced these forms to elementary motions and forces in which the same mechanical laws accounted for all change. Gone was the kinship between the human logos and anything in nature (Jonas, 1966, pp. 66–70; 1974, pp. 51–65). Gone also was the hierarchy in which some objects were nobler than others.

The realm of living things in general and human nature in particular were not exempted from the mechanistic model, but for some time they were spared its full implications. While this model could explain the actual functioning of organisms, its use to explain the generation of present states from antecedent states—an extension that was delayed in the case of the physical world because of its theological dangers—was hindered by the very nature of organisms, whose genesis and development appeared to result from the unfolding of the pattern imbedded in the species, and thus indicated formal causation rather than mechanical laws. The origins of the species themselves required something other than mechanical laws since their complexity entailed enormous odds for their chance production (Jonas, 1966, pp. 38–42). In other words, something of substantial form and rational order remained in the development of the organism, however much its functions could be explained by mechanics. This, of course, changed with the doctrine of the evolution of species. Once the first primitive life forms were spontaneously produced by inorganic matter, the species and their patterns could be understood as the product of the random play of variations resulting from the disequilibrium of antecedent states and proceeding according to mechanical laws (Jonas, 1966, pp. 42–45).

This is a familiar story, but Jonas emphasizes three implications of the mechanistic worldview. The first is what he calls the "ontology of death": in contrast to the ancients for whom death is the limit of knowledge, the living world is now knowable only as matter,that is, as lifeless. The body, therefore, is intelligible only as corpse (Jonas, 1966, pp. 9–12). Jonas does not mention the significance for modern medicine of this way of treating the body, but I discuss his ongoing argument that organic life must be understood as purposive, and the body as living body, in the following section.

The second implication is the banishment of value and teleology from the world. In addition to the uniformity of all entities, which leveled the premodern value hierarchy of beings, the quantitative equivalence of cause and effect together with the axiom of the constancy of matter and energy ruled out both extraphysical efficient causes (e.g., divine action or human purpose) and final causes of any kind (Jonas, 1974, p. 66). As a result, "[n]ature is not a place where one can look for ends. Efficient cause knows no preference of outcomes: the complete absence of final causes means that nature is indifferent to distinctions of value. It cannot be thwarted because it has nothing to achieve" (Jonas, 1974, p. 69). Jonas is quick to point out that these conclusions are are not logically necessary but are metaphysical corollaries of the conceptual framework of modern science and its a priori presuppositions.[5] More is said about the underlying metaphysics and Jonas's postcritical alternative in the following section. Here I only underscore that what holds for the physical world holds as well for the organic world when both are assumed under the mechanistic model. If the structures of life (i.e, species) are merely the product of random variations resulting in an equilibrium between organism and environment, then there is no fixed telos of human nature, and thus no stable conception or image of the human to be derived from nature (Jonas, 1966, pp. 45–47).

The result of the loss of teleology is nihilism. "With the rejection of teleology from the system of natural causes, nature, itself purposeless, ceased to provide any sanction to possible human purposes" (Jonas, 1966, pp. 214–215). Without a hierarchy of beings or an immanent finality, all natural events, while necessary with respect to cause, are accidental with respect to value. The result is that nature (including human nature) is without a norm to determine which technological interventions, if any, are justifiable. "If nature sanctions nothing, then it permits everything. Whatever man does to it, he does not violate an immanent integrity, to which it and all its works have lost title. In a nature that is its own perpetual accident, each thing can as well be other than it is without being any the less natural" (Jonas, 1974, p. 70). In the absence of any norm inherent in nature, the only remaining source of norms is that which in the Cartesian framework escapes the mechanistic reduction: the will. This leads Jonas to conclude that the heir of Descartes and Darwin is Nietzsche.[6] Since there is no value or end to discover in nature, the will must create values and ends (Jonas, 1966, p. 215). As the sole subject, the will confronts nature as mere object. No longer enjoying with it the kinship of the logos, the subject who wills is estranged from the world, which he now meets as an object for use at best and an alien power that is indifferent to his concerns at worst.[7] Either way, the will is a will to power, subjecting nature to human use or countering its indifference to human concerns. In both cases, nihilism gives birth to technological mastery.

In short, Jonas narrates a version of the dialectic of Enlightment thesis, according to which "the very same movement that put us in possession of the powers that have now to be regulated by norms—the movement of modern knowledge called science—has by a necessary complementarity eroded the foundations from which norms could be derived; it has destroyed the very idea of norm as such" (Jonas, 1984, p. 22).

The third implication of the new worldview of modern science pertains to the nature of technology itself. Jonas argues that even though it was roughly two centuries before the new science directly influenced technology, the latter was implicit in mechanistic science, so that its eventual connection with science was neither accidental nor simply an application of science. The conceptual analysis of motion made possible by Descartes' analytical geometry and later by the infinitesimal calculus of Newton and Leibniz reduced complex motions to their component simple parts, thus permitting the isolation and quantification of factors essential to the experimental method, which in turn became the means to knowledge (Jonas, 1974, p. 63). Science is therefore inherently technological in a twofold sense.

> The very conception of reality that underlay and was fostered by the rise of modern science, i.e., the new concept of *nature*, con-

tained manipulability at its theoretical core and, in the form of experiment, involved actual manipulation in the investigative process. . . . Technology was thus implied as a *possibility* in the metaphysics, and trained as a *practice* in the procedures of modern science. (Jonas, 1974, p. 48)

Put differently, "understanding of this sort is itself a kind of making or remaking of its objects, and this is the deepest cause for the technological applicability of modern science" (Jonas, 1966, p. 202). This complex and interdependent relation between science and technology determines both the formal and the material character of modern technology. Formally, the relation of science and technology involves the dynamics of endless progress. Science as theory makes the experiment possible by its view of nature. The experiment intervenes into nature in order to gain knowledge about the latter. The knowledge thus gained eventually leads to the large-scale enhancements and manipulations of nature involved in modern technology, which themselves lead to further theoretical insights and to the tools to carry out more effective experimentation (Jonas, 1966, pp. 204–205). In short, "a mutual feedback operates between science and technology," a feedback that involves mutual dependence and requires the endless progress of technology. More generally, modern technology is characterized by a fluidity of ends and a circular relation in which new technology designed as novel means to existing ends continually creates and imposes new ends (Jonas, 1979, p. 35).[8] It follows that progress is "not at all a mere option" offered by modern technology "but an inherent drive" that belongs to its formal dynamics (Jonas, 1979, p. 35). Technology, whether by design or default, is utopian in form.

If scientific understanding is itself according to Jonas a making or remaking of its objects, it follows that the most salient material characteristic of technology is its artificial character: technology is the triumph of making. In fact, making comprises for Jonas the essence of technology in the Heideggerian sense, namely its mode of manifesting reality. It is therefore not surprising that Jonas describes the progress of technology in terms of its increasing artificiality. At first, technology simply facilitated the production of familiar objects that met common human needs. At this stage art still imitated nature (Jonas, 1979, pp. 38–39). This changed with modern chemistry. While mechanics uses natural materials and forces, chemistry alters the substances of nature, creates synthetic substances and, in the case of molecular engineering, redesigns the very patterns of nature. "Man steps into nature's shoes, and from utilizing and exploiting he advances to creating. . . . Artificiality enters the heart of matter" (Jonas, 1974, p. 77). But while chemistry still deals with material found in natural experience, electricity is an abstract object discovered by science and, insofar as it is a manipulable force, is an artificial creation (Jonas, 1974, p. 78). Electronic technology is yet further removed from nature. With its advent, technology is no longer "nature supplemented, imitated, improved, transformed," but rather results in a *"transnature* of human making."* The objects of electronic technology are wholly artificial, and it serves artificial ends far removed from natural human needs (Jonas, 1974, p. 79; 1979, p. 40).[9]

It should be clear now why for Jonas molecular biology is not only the last but also the most ominous frontier of technology. While Jonas remained deeply concerned about the effects of human making on non-human nature, the development of genetic and other forms of biological engineering harbor a possible future in which making turns on and threatens to consume the maker himself. "But man himself has been added to the objects of technology. *Homo faber* is turning on himself and gets ready to make over the maker of all the rest" (Jonas, 1984, p. 18). Here technology seems for Jonas to reveal most clearly and decisively the dialectic that constitutes it, for here the power of the modern subject over all that is external realizes itself as power over that subject himself.[10] The very technology that began as the product of the subject's control over the world now threatens to turn the subject himself into a product by means of behavior control, genetic engineering, and elimination of aging. But if this kind of rational control is destined to recoil back on the controller himself, the impending final stage of the technological revolution urgently calls for an alternative conception of the human.

> If and when *that* revolution occurs, if technological power is really going to tinker with the elemental keys on which life will have to play its melody in generations of men to come . . . then a reflection on what is humanly desirable and what should determine the choice—a reflection, in short, on the image of man, becomes an imperative more urgent than any ever inflicted on the understanding of mortal man. (Jonas, 1979, p. 41)

But of course, the urgent imperative of reflection on the image of the human runs up against the two factors described above: nihilism and "the inherently 'utopian' drift of our actions under the conditions of modern technology" (Jonas, 1984, p. 21).

I began this section by claiming that for Jonas, Descartes developed the view of reality that the Baconian project required in order to succeed. I have pointed out the nihilistic implications of this view of reality and have described both the formal dynamics of progress and the material emphasis on making, culminating in the remaking of the maker, that for Jonas characterize modern technology. Now is the time to draw these observations into the critique of utopia. Here Jonas seeks to identify an arc of thought stretching from Bacon to Marx to contemporary technology, and which is summarized in the utopian claim that humanity is yet to be realized in its fullness, a fullness to be brought about in large part by technology. The following analysis reconstructs a narrative that is nowhere explicit in Jonas's texts but that I believe is central to understanding his major task. This task is to challenge the claim that humanity is yet to be realized and to oppose to it an anti-utopian ethic that is the topic of the following section.

Jonas and his utopian opponents share a common first premise. Both agree that in the transition from the view that human nature is grounded in fixed essences to the view that human nature emerges in the flux of becoming, the good has become historical and vulnerable to the powers of modern technology. This departure from the relation between human beings and the good in antiquity is fundamental and irreversible. "It is in this context that responsibility can become dominant in morality. The Platonic eros, directed at eternity, at the nontemporal, is not responsible for its object. For this 'is' and never 'becomes.' What time cannot affect and to which nothing can happen is an object not of responsibility but of emulation" (Jonas, 1984, p. 125). On this point Jonas and the modern ethic of utopia are in agreement, and to that extent they both depart from the ethics of antiquity. But Jonas departs from the utopians when they transform the ancient ideal of perfection into a historical goal that humans are responsible for bringing about. Jonas finds a gradual emergence of this transformation in western thought. While present in a naive and proleptic sense in Bacon, its explicit formulation in moral theory begins with Kant, for whom the highest good is to be progressively approximated in a time series. But this good remains a regulative idea that is not brought about by human causality in history. For Hegel the regulative idea becomes constitutive and time becomes the medium of its realization, but it occurs without the conscious willing of the human agents through whom it is realized. Only with Marx is there *"responsibility for the historical future in collusion with history's own dynamism . . ."* (Jonas, 1984, p. 127). With Marx also the past becomes a mere stepping-stone to the present which in turn is a mere stepping stone to the future. Like other forms of modern utopianism, Marxism's

> resolute secular eschatology entails a conception of human events
> that radically demotes to provisional status all that goes before,

> stripping it of its independent validity and at best making it the vehicle for reaching the promised state of things that is yet to come—a means to the future end which alone is worthy in itself. (Jonas, 1984, pp. 16–17)

The result in the case of Marxism is the twofold commitment to the true human who is yet to come and to the technology that is to bring it about (Jonas, 1984, pp. 154–157, 198–201). The exemplar of this combination is Ernst Bloch's "ontology of the 'not yet,'" the major facet of his "principle of hope" against which Jonas directs his "principle of responsibility." While Jonas is preoccupied with its Marxist version, this twofold commitment marks the point at which any version of the Baconian project becomes an explicit vision for a future humanity. Hence in addition to Bloch's (and Bacon's) vision of a humanity freed from the ceaseless round of toil, we may add the visions of biomedical utopians who seek to enhance human traits, forestall or reverse the processes of aging, or alter human behavior.

But Marxism is not the culmination of the process. While Marxist utopianism does not spell out its utopia in detail, it retains the assumption that human beings know the direction and goal of progress. (The same applies to the biomedical utopians.) An element of the regulative or constitutive ideas of its Kantian and Hegelian forerunners persists in Marxism and spares the latter from nihilism. But this element is lost in the case of technology per se, which could therefore be viewed as a form of utopia without a metanarrative. "With technology's having seized power—a revolution this, planned by no one, totally anonymous and irresistible—the dynamism has taken on aspects not contained in any earlier idea of it, and not foreseeable by any theory, Marxist or other" (Jonas, 1984, pp. 127–128). In other words, the dynamics of modern technology overtake the human effort to realize—even to formulate—an objective ideal in history. Technology thus overcomes the last efforts to wrest a substantive good from the flux of the world of Descartes and Darwin, as technological progress itself becomes, by default, the de facto ideal. The result is that modern technology is at once both utopian and nihilistic. It is utopian since it clings to the notion that humanity is yet to be realized. It is nihilistic since its imperviousness to any substantive ideal leaves it beyond good and evil. In the case of biomedicine, efforts to spell out the utopia modern medicine will usher in are no longer needed; it is enough simply to keep pushing the frontiers of life extension, genetic control, forestalling of aging, and so forth. Modern technology, including biomedicine, moves toward no ideal to be realized, but simply keeps moving forward.

Now, *techne* in the form of modern technology has turned into an infinite forward-thrust of the race, its most significant enterprise, in whose permanent, self-transcending advance to ever greater things the vocation of man tends to be seen, and whose success of maximal control over things and himself appears as the consummation of his destiny. (Jonas, 1984, p. 9)

The making leads toward no goal, and the power is no longer the power of a subject to realize a goal. Power itself is the goal, and this kind of power is power over the subject.[11]

AN ETHIC OF RESPONSIBILITY

It should now be clear what kind of an ethic Jonas believes the technological era demands. First, nihilism can be overcome only by a form of objective good that can impose upon the otherwise arbitrary will obligations or duties regarding the exercise of the powers of technology and their restraint. Second, utopianism can be overcome only if Jonas can show why humanity is not still to be realized. And since Jonas precludes a return to premodern ethics, he will have to provide a conception of the human that confers normative significance on humanity-as-it-is while also taking account of the historical nature of human beings and the evolution of human nature from previous forms of life. Such an ethic, therefore, will have to develop a conception of humanity-as-it-is (not as something yet to be realized) as an objective good that imposes an obligation on the human will which through technology has power over this objective good. The chief question, then, is this: Is there some feature of humanity-as-it-is by virtue of which the latter can be shown to be an objective good which, precisely as an objective good, imposes an obligation to ensure its present and future existence against actions that might radically alter or destroy it?

To answer this question affirmatively, Jonas will have to show how human beings are responsible for what comes under their power. Only if what is under their power (namely, humanity-as-it-is) can be shown to be an objective good can it make them responsible for it in the sense indicated in the previous paragraph. Jonas will therefore have to show how that which is subject to our power can nevertheless have the same kind of objective claim on our wills that the exalted objects of contemplation once had. In language that calls to mind Emmanuel Levinas's ethics of alterity, Jonas notes the difference between the ethics of responsibility, whose object is vulnerable yet not appropriated, and the ancient ethics of the transcendent good, whose object is self-sufficient yet capable of being appropriated.[12]

> [T]he object of *responsibility* is emphatically the perishable *qua* perishable. Yet in spite of this condition which it shares with myself, it is more unshareably an "other" to me than any of the transcendent objects of classical ethics: "other" not as the surpassing better, but as nothing-but-itself in its own right, and without *this* otherness being meant to be bridged by a qualitative assimilation on my part or on its part. Precisely this otherness takes possession of my responsibility, and no appropriation is intended here. Yet just this far from "perfect" object, entirely contingent in its facticity, perceived precisely in its perishability, indigence, and insecurity, must have the power to move me through its sheer existence . . . to place my person at its service, free of all appetite for appropriation. (Jonas, 1984, p. 87)

As a paradigm of the moral life, this description indicates that responsibility will differ from modern ethics, which replaced emulation of the transcendent good with the reciprocity of independent adults as the paradigm of morality. That over which I have power exists not in a reciprocal but in an assymetrical relation to me. For this reason Jonas, as I show below, borrowing from Hannah Arendt and Max Weber, respectively, substitutes the parent and the statesman for the reciprocity of independent adults as exemplars of the moral life (Arendt, 1958, pp. 246–247; Weber, 1958, pp. 115–128).

The powers of technology force us, as we have seen, to raise the question of the normative status of humanity itself, which it is now under our power to alter or destroy. Due to the expanded range of action under modern technology, many of our actions, ranging from destruction of the biosphere to genetic engineering, have real or potential effects on the very nature and existence of future human beings, as well as their quality of life. Jonas is convinced that moral feeling supports the requirement to ensure a future for humanity. But a future of what kind and a humanity of what description? And how is feeling to respond to the reflection which in all sincerity questions any moral claim of future humanity? The first question points to the need for a rationally defensible conception of the normatively human; the second question calls for a response to the view that only present human beings have moral claims or that the very notion of duties to future human beings is based on a confusion.

Jonas begins by opposing something like the following view. We have no knowledge of any essential nature of humanity, and even if we did a basic consequentialist principle would tell us that distant and uncertain threats should not outweigh proximate and more certain benefits. Since we are relatively certain about the advantages to be derived from increased economic output or genetic engineering, and since the threats they pose are uncertain and in any case would occur only in the distant future, there is no moral reason not to proceed with them. In opposition to this view or something like it, Jonas concedes that all predictive knowledge is conjectural but denies that this supports the consequentialist position. First, precisely because it alerts us to what is at stake in our technological ambitions, conjectural knowledge may serve an epistemological role in determining what is to be preserved from those ambitions. For "it is an anticipated *distortion* of man that helps us to detect that in the normative conception of man which is to be preserved from it. And we need the *threat* to the image of man—and rather specific kinds of threat—to assure ourselves of his true image by the very recoil from those threats" (Jonas, 1984, pp. 26–27). Such conjectural knowledge, by telling us what there is to fear about the effects of our actions, serves the heuristic purpose of helping us to discover what is the normatively human. That such predictive knowledge is conjectural and uncertain is no hindrance to this purely heuristic function.

Second, uncertainty may itself be the cause of a principle that opposes the consequentialist line of reasoning. Here Jonas develops an ethic of risk or wager in two steps. He begins with his own consequential consideration, invoking the irreversibility and cumulativity of technological action: if supremely evil effects occur we will not be able to correct them. Next he argues that making use of our inherited constitution in order to act in a way that puts that very constitution at risk involves a performative self-contradiction. Since this is a version of the liar's paradox, I will call it the "improver's paradox." If one indicates a willingness to put our evolutionary heritage at risk, one disparages that heritage as lacking and thereby disqualifies oneself as a product of that heritage for the task of improving it. But if one affirms oneself as capable of improving this heritage, one affirms the worth of one's inherited constitution, which therefore must not be tampered with (Jonas, 1984, p. 33). Jonas's purpose in pointing out the paradox is simply to show that there is a condition for the creative steering of destiny that is incommensurable with the order of things subject to calculations of risk and benefit or gain and loss involved in such steering. The argument reveals that among the stakes risked in the game, there is one of metaphysical rank (physical as its origins may be), an "absolute" which, as a supreme and vulnerable trust, lays upon us the supreme duty to preserve it intact. This duty is beyond comparison superior to all the injunctions and wishes of a meliorism in the peripheral zones, and, where it is concerned, the question is no longer one of weighing chances of finite profit and loss but one of contraposing the risk of infinite loss against chances of finite gains. No weighing (e.g. of probability differentials) has still a place between these incommensurables. (Jonas, 1984, pp. 33–34)

Both of Jonas's arguments against the consequentialist position summarized above use the uncertainty of our knowledge of the effects of our actions to identify something that is not subject to consequential weighing. If a contemplated action of ours puts at risk a good whose value is incommensurable with other goods to be realized by that action, our uncertainty over the outcome of the action works against the consequentialist argument above. Such risks may be acceptable in cases of supreme emergency, but not to achieve the melioristic gains at which modern technology aims. But there are problems with both arguments. A heuristic use of conjecture can at most present us with candidates for a normative conception of the human; it is insufficient to justify any such candidate. But without a justifiable conception, the consequentialist argument still stands. Moreover, the improver's paradox applies to actions that would use the capacity to steer destiny in ways that would risk destroying that capacity either by the loss from the earth of those who bear that capacity or by turning its bearers into automatons. But it is difficult to know what interventions would fall under these descriptions. It would seem to apply directly only to the most extreme actions: a large-scale nuclear endeavor, germ-line enhancement on a massive scale, or advanced neurosurgical procedures. (Given the dynamics of technology, Jonas could be arguing that even the early stages of environmental degradation, germ-line therapy, and use of neurology for behavioral control risk destroying the relevant human capacity.) The improver's paradox has two additional problems that Jonas himself mentions. One is that it has nothing to say to the nihilist who neither disparages the evolutionary heritage nor claims superior qualification due to it, but simply asserts that since nature sanctions nothing, it permits whatever the playing impulse combined with technological mastery wishes to create (Jonas, 1984, p. 33). The other problem is that the argument assumes what is yet to be proved: that we are responsible for there being future human beings at all. It will turn out that Jonas's major argument claims to provide the solution to both of these problems.

That we are responsible for future human beings who will be affected by our present actions and that such responsibility obligates us to ensure the existence of future humanity in a yet-to-be-defined normative sense is, as we noted above, central to Jonas's argument against the consequentialist view that the future existence of humanity could without moral condemnation be risked in order to supply the needs and wants of present human beings or to improve the human condition. There seems to be, as Jonas observes, something intuitive about such a responsibility, but arguments to justify it have foundered. Those who would assign rights to future persons face the problem that rights imply already-existing persons who are capable of claiming them and suffering violations of them. "But the ethic we seek is concerned with just this not-yet-existent; and *its* principle of responsibility must be independent of any idea of a right and therefore also of a reciprocity . . ." (Jonas, 1984, p. 39). Of course, infants are not capable of claiming rights, but we generally extend to them the right to live. So perhaps the notion of reciprocity is the problem, and we can simply extend a nonreciprocal right to exist to future persons on the same grounds as we do for infants, namely because they are our progeny. But this will not work. The extension of rights to infants follows from the responsibility of the cause for the effect it has brought about. That which has not yet been brought about in the first place has no right to exist (Jonas, 1984, pp. 39–40). Changing tactics, one may argue that since there will in any case be future persons, we are obligated to ensure that they will have no grounds for complaint about the conditions of their existence. But first of all, there need not be future persons at all. A sincere pessimist could argue that the continuation of the human race is just not worth it in light of the conditions under which future persons will live. Moreover, this argument establishes the approval or disapproval of future persons as the source of our obligations to them. But we do not know what future persons will approve—it is possible that they would praise us for depriving them of what we know as the dignity and vocation of the human (Jonas, 1984, p. 41). One might think of the gratitude future persons might have toward us for programming the equivalent of a Nozickian pleasure machine into the brain or germ line after we had finally identified the appropriate neurotransmitters or genes and developed the techniques—assuming they would still be capable of gratitude.

The failure of these attempts to establish the principle of responsibility for ensuring a future humanity of a certain description leads Jonas to his most innovative, ambitious and controversial move.[13] This involves his claim that "there is . . . an *unconditional duty* for mankind to exist" (Jonas, 1984, p. 37). The source of the duty is an ought that stands above both ourselves and future human beings. It is therefore not their rights or wishes but "their *duty* over which we have to watch, namely, their duty to be truly human: thus over their *capacity* for this duty . . . which *we* could possibly rob them of with the alchemy of our 'utopian' technology" (Jonas, 1984, p. 42). This leads to a rule, namely "that no condition of future descendents of humankind should be permitted to arise which contradicts the reason why the existence of mankind is mandatory at all" (Jonas, 1984, p. 43). Jonas therefore avoids the problems associated with future individuals: the ought refers not to identifiable future individuals but to the idea of humanity, which stands over both us and the future humans over whom technology gives us power.

> With this imperative, we are, strictly speaking, not responsible to the future human individuals but to the *idea* of Man. . . . It is this ontological imperative, emanating from the idea of Man, which stands behind the prohibition of a *va-banque* gamble with mankind. Only the idea of Man, by telling us *why* there should be men, tells us also *how* they should be. (Jonas, 1984, p. 43)

In his effort to avoid the problems and paradoxes of future individuals, Jonas proposes nothing less than a moral version of the ontological argument: that the very idea of humanity makes the existence of humanity an imperative. If this argument succeeds, it will identify a conception of the human that tells us both why humanity ought to be and how—that is, in what form or by virtue of what feature(s)—humanity ought to be. It will thereby set a limit to those technologies that in their quest for control over necessity and improvement of human nature threaten the existence of humanity so conceived.

This argument stands or falls on two premises, one formal and the other material. The formal premise holds that the only thing that of itself grounds a valid claim to being is the good, provided that the latter is genuinely objective and not simply in the willing or desiring of a subject.

> For the good or valuable, when it is this of itself and not just by the grace of someone's desiring, needing, or choosing, is by its very concept a thing whose being possible entails the demand for its being or becoming actual and thus turns into an "ought" when a will is present which can hear the demand and translate it into action. (Jonas, 1984, p. 79; cf. also p. 48)

Jonas does not argue for but rather assumes this premise, which is nevertheless controversial. The second premise is that purposiveness is such an objective good and thus becomes an ought, and its being or becoming actual becomes a duty for an agent when it depends on his or her action (or abstention). The argument for this premise proceeds in three steps. First, Jonas argues for the objectivity of purposiveness which, in contrast to the Cartesian view of reality, he finds in nature itself and not only in human willing. But while its having purposes indicates that nature has ends and therefore values, merely having values does not make them valuable, that is, good. So the second step is to argue that the mere capacity to have purposes is good in itself. The third and final step is to argue that our primary responsibility is to human purposiveness.

The argument that nature has purposes is the crucial part of the material premise in Jonas's argument, one that he spent much of his career trying to establish. He first argued for this premise in the form of a phenomenology of the living body in which one may hear echoes of Edmund Husserl and Heidegger.[14] Against the dualist notion of a pure consciousness set over against pure extension, Jonas argues from the phenomenon of causality for the coincidence of inwardness and outwardness in the living body. In opposition to Hume and Kant, whose assumption that perception as receptivity is the only mode in which the external world is given led them to view causality as a mental addition to the prime givenness of reality, Jonas shows how causality "has its seat in the *effort* I must make to overcome the resistance of worldly matter in my acting and to resist the impact of worldly matter upon myself." Causality, therefore, "is rooted in just the point of actual, live 'transcendence' of the self, the point where inwardness actively transcends itself into the outward and continues itself into it with its actions" (Jonas, 1966, p. 23).[15] Inwardness here is of course purposiveness: inwardness transcends itself and continues itself into the outward precisely in the causative force of purpose, which meets the resistance of the world. The living body thus transgresses the divisions established by the ontic separation of consciousness and extension. And because the living body is given not as a content of consciousness but in its active engagement with the world, it quite naturally extrapolates from its own experience into the whole of reality. In the case of causality, "advancing from my body, nay, myself advancing bodily, I build up . . . the dynamic image . . . of a world of force and resistance, action and inertia, cause and effect" (Jonas, 1966, p. 23).

There are, however, two barriers to taking this phenomenology as an ontology of living things in general and thus securing the ontological grounding of purpose. First, phenomenology ascribes the inwardness of purpose to the living body per se as a striving organism. But our own awareness of purpose, from which we extrapolate to organisms in general, is always a conscious awareness (Jonas, 1984, p. 65). On what grounds does Jonas extend purposiveness beyond those beings whose testimony confirms it; that is, beyond conscious beings? Without this extrapolation, of course, the argument that purposiveness is confined to human willing gains force. But is such an extrapolation justified? Second, materialism also claims to overcome dualism, in this case by bringing the testimony of the living body under its own principles. In response to the first barrier, Jonas argues that "the living body is the archetype of the concrete, and being *my* body it is, in its immediacy of inwardness and outwardness in one, the *only* given concrete of experience in general" (Jonas, 1966, p. 24). Phenomenology works from concrete experience, but if my body, the body I concretely experience, exhibits certain qualities by virtue of its being a living body, then it is appropriate to understand the living in general from this perspective. This leads Jonas to argue that purposiveness resides even in metabolism. Like a machine, the organism consists wholly of its parts, but unlike the machine it consists wholly in its own performance in which it builds up and continually replaces the parts of the machine. "Metabolism thus is the constant becoming of the machine itself—and this becoming itself is a performance of the machine" (Jonas, 1966, p. 76, n.13). Herein lies the problem with materialism. In metabolism the organism both is and is not identical to its matter. At any point it consists wholly of its matter. Yet if it were identified with its matter, it would be dead. Moreover, it is not identical with the successive stages of its matter since it exists whole and complete in each stage. Rather, its identity consists in its performance or self-integration carried out in the constant exchange of matter with its surroundings (Jonas, 1966, pp. 79–80; 1974, pp. 190–192). Performance or self-integration in turn implies purposiveness, which therefore characterizes the organism as such and distinguishes it from nonliving reality.

> *Teleology* comes in where the continuous identity of being is not assured by mere inertial persistence of a substance [as in inorganic reality], but is continually executed by something *done*, and by something which *has* to be done in order to stay on at all: it is a matter of to-be-or-not-to-be whether what is to be done *is* done. Now to an entity that carries on its existence by way of constant regenerative activity we impute *concern*. (Jonas, 1974, p. 197)

Like Heidegger's Dasein, the being of the organism is continually realized against the possibility of its not-being, which gives its being the character of care or concern. The problem with materialism and its denial of any purposiveness outside the will "lay in denying organic reality its principle and most obvious characteristic, namely, that it exhibits in each individual existence a striving of its own for existence and fulfillment, or the fact of life's willing itself" (Jonas, 1966, p. 61).

Nevertheless, as Richard Zaner has argued, Jonas's extrapolation trades on a shift from a phenomenology of *my* living body to a philosophical analysis of organism in general (Zaner, 1981, pp. 14–21). The appeal to the active engagement with the world I experience in exerting force stands on phenomenological grounds, but the argument that organic life in general exhibits the same feature of striving must appeal to other kinds of evidence and to theory. However, I believe Jonas eventually abandoned this approach. In his later work the phenomenological testimony of the subject is validated and extended to organic life in general not by extrapolation but by (negative) metaphysical arguments. Now Jonas's argument against materialism seeks to vindicate the testimony of the acting subject by showing how theories that deny it are incoherent and are not necessary even to preserve the integrity of the mechanical laws of nature. This testimony is that thought has causative force both inside and outside itself, namely in the acting body. "But with the determination of the body, which hence continues forth into the surrounding world, subjective purposes acquire an objective role in the fabric of events: that fabric, therefore, that is, physical nature, must have room for such interventions by a nonphysical agency" (Jonas, 1984, p. 64). Materialism cannot accept such a causative force, so it seeks either to rule out psychical interference altogether on grounds of the constancy of the laws of nature or to deny any causative force to the psychical as an epiphenomenon. In response to the first, Jonas denies that the constancy laws are necessarily unconditional and that they can be applied so rigorously. His response to the second employs several arguments, one of which is that epiphenomenalism requires an effect (the epiphenomenon) that occurs without expenditure of any causal energy and that itself has no effect. Both of these requirements contradict the materialist account of causality and leave it an utter mystery why something with no causal power and thus no efficacy for survival would have evolved in the first place (Jonas, 1984, pp. 207–212).[16]

If materialism fails to thwart the subjective (i.e., phenomenological) testimony of purposiveness, can Jonas's broader task of extending a purposive element beyond beings with consciousness succeed? Does it make sense to attribute concern or purposiveness to beings that lack consciousness? Jonas's argument here is also negative and is explicitly metaphysical. It shows that the alternative view, that such subjectivity began with conscious beings, is untenable because it requires either a theory of ingression in which subjectivity seized upon a certain configuration of matter (i.e., the brain) in order to ingress into nature at a particular point, or a theory of emergence in which subjectivity emerges with the suitable material conditions. The first view presupposes the prior existence of subjectivity and therefore invites all the problems of dualism. In the second view, it is unclear how subjectivity as a qualitative leap is compatible with the gradual transition that characterizes the material substratum from which it emerges, or how the new level can constrain or codetermine the substratum (Jonas, 1984, pp. 66–69). The only solution to these problems is to affirm a principle of continuity in which we "let ourselves be *instructed by what is highest and richest concerning everything beneath it*" (Jonas, 1984, p. 69). Following this principle, the subjective purposiveness we know in ourselves gradually shades off into sensitivity and appetition without a focused subject as we descend the scale of being. But nowhere does striving disappear altogether. "On the strength of the evidence of life (which we of its stock in whom it has come to know itself should be the last to deny), we say therefore that purpose in general is indigenous to nature" (Jonas, 1984, pp. 73–74).

Nature, then, has purposes and therefore has values. If Jonas's argument is valid he has established the first of the three steps in his material premise. But since for any particular purpose the fact of it comes before the good it seeks, that good is relative to the purpose and is not a good in itself. Nature can not legitimize its purposes merely by having them. But the situation is different, Jonas argues, for purposiveness itself. "We can regard the mere *capacity* to *have* any purposes at all as a good-in-itself, of which we grasp with intuitive certainty that it is infinitely superior to any purposelessness of being" (Jonas, 1984, p. 80). In affirming itself over against nonbeing, being makes its difference from nonbeing the basic value (i.e., its difference from nonbeing is not a matter of indifference). To say no to being or even to the value difference of being that being affirms over against the value indifference of nonbeing (or of value-indifferent being) is to affirm value difference and thus purposiveness (Jonas, 1984, p. 81). However, Jonas realizes that the intrinsic goodness of purposiveness is finally an intuition, and its affirmation "a matter of ultimate metaphysical choice" (Jonas, 1984, p. 80). It must be so for the following reason: while a denial of purposiveness as good (e.g., a claim that being would have been better if it had been utterly indifferent) itself expresses purpose precisely because, as a denial, it is not indifferent, nothing can logically force one from a state of utter indifference as to whether value difference (i.e., purposiveness) is to be preferred to value indifference. Jonas himself seems to recognize this problem (Jonas, 1974, pp. 87–88, n. 4).

Assuming such a metaphysical choice, purposiveness is therefore a good in itself. This is the point of the second step in Jonas's material premise. But he has not yet secured his principle of responsibility. In human beings, the goodness of purposiveness is not affirmed blindly by being but must be affirmed by the will. But why should not the case be for human beings as it is for all other creatures, namely that any exercise of purpose affirms purposiveness, so that (in the case of humans) all willing—even the willing of the self-destruction or radical alteration of humanity—would be justified as the fulfilment of natural purpose? Jonas argues that while every purpose is a value, human beings distinguish ends as worthy and unworthy independently of inclination. In the "primordial phenomenon of *demanding*," the good as worthy apart from the inclinations addresses the will as an ought "in the situation where the realization or preservation of *this* good by *this* subject is a concrete issue" (Jonas, 1984, p. 84). Jonas thus appeals to a Kantian fact of obligation that stands over against inclination but which, in contrast to Kant, commands as an objective good and not as the moral law.

> Not duty itself is the object; not the moral law motivates moral action, but the appeal of a possible good-in-itself in the world, which confronts my will and demands to be heard—*in accordance with* the moral law. To grant that appeal a hearing *is* precisely what the moral law commands. . . . It makes my duty what insight has shown to be, of itself, worthy of being and in need of my acting. (Jonas, 1984, p. 85)

But for a good in itself to affect me in this way, I must be receptive to it. As we saw above, this requires a receptivity not to the intrinsic claim of an exalted object, but to that of an object over which I have power. In Jonas's terms, I feel responsible for that which has come under my power. "The demand of the object in the unassuredness of its existence, on the one hand, and the conscience of power in the guilt of its causality, on the other hand, conjoin in the affirmative feeling of responsibility on the part of a self that anyway and always must actively encroach on the being of things" (Jonas, 1984, p. 93). In other words, the right-to-be of the object and its vulnerability to my power affect sensibility in the form of a feeling of responsibility for the object, a feeling that includes reverence for and a readiness to act on behalf of the object.[17]

Here the paradigms of the parent and the statesman alert us to the the primacy of responsibility over notions of ethics that assume reciprocity. Parental responsibility in particular constitutes the archetype of responsibility: the newborn brought about by my causative action is, as now existing, an unquestioned good in itself while, as still becoming, it is also vulnerable and indigent and dependent on my action to realize itself. "Utmost facticity of 'thisness,' utmost right thereto, and utmost fragility of being meet here together" (Jonas, 1984, p. 135).

I have now discussed both the objectivity of purposiveness and the sense in which purposiveness is a good in itself and its realization and preservation an ought for human beings. The third step in the material premise of Jonas's argument is the primacy of responsibility for human purposiveness. Only human beings can have responsibility for the purposes of other beings. This capacity means that they can in a unique manner include fellow human beings in their responsibility. To be responsible for fellow humans is to be responsible for those who are themselves responsible. This reversibility, according to which the objects of our responsibility are themselves responsible subjects, means that their purposiveness can become our purpose in a uniquely kindred manner (Jonas, 1984, pp. 98–99). But in what sense does the purposiveness of other humans become our responsibility? It certainly can not mean that their individual purposes become ours, since these will differ from ours and especially since those for whom we are responsible include future human beings whose purposes we do not know. What we can uniquely include in our own responsibility is the responsibility of others: their very capacity for exercising responsibility according to the demands of situations that call for it. This is the duty of future humans over which we have to watch, namely their "duty to be truly human," as we noted above, which stands above them and ourselves, who could deprive them of it (cf. Jonas, 1984, p. 42). This is the "idea of Man," which by telling us *why* there should be human beings (because of the objective goodness of responsibility as the highest form of purposiveness) tells us *how* they should be (namely, capable of being responsible) (Jonas, 1984, p. 43). Hence the first object of responsibility is "the possibility of there being responsibility in the world," the possibility, that is, of there being "mere *candidates* for a moral order" (Jonas, 1984, pp. 99, 10). Responsibility for the natural order that sustains responsible beings follows accordingly.

Once again, the paradigmatic role of the parent and the statesman prepare us for understanding this seemingly abstract responsibility for responsibility. Both are responsible for a future of their children and communities that lies beyond their knowledge and control. In fact, the ultimate object of commitment in both cases is to the autonomous causality of the life under their care, a causality the future self-assertion of which the parent or statesman not only can not control but are not responsible for at all. If this is so, "the intent of the responsibility must be not so much to determine as to enable, that is, to prepare and keep the capacity for itself in those to come intact, never foreclosing the future exercise of responsibility by them" (Jonas, 1984, p. 107).

If we are responsible primarily for there continuing to be agents capable of responding to the demands of new situations rather than for quality of future life or an ideal future state, the implications for utopianism are clear. Insofar as human beings are responsible, they are not still to be realized. "Our summary thesis is clear: the future (not to speak of its essential unknowability) is no less, but also no more, 'itself' and for its own sake than was any portion of the past. . . . Mankind, since it exists . . . is always 'already there' and never still to be brought about" (Jonas, 1984, pp. 109–110). Because of the freedom entailed in responsibility and the uniqueness of future situations in which it will be exercised, "man will indeed be always new and different from all before him, but never more 'genuine'" (Jonas, 1984, p. 201).

In short, the normatively human is in the first place responsibility itself, which has become the object of our responsibility because it is threatened by our capacity to destroy the conditions for human life and by our potential power to remake the maker through genetic and neurological engineering. The argument for responsibility, however, is not merely an academic moral argument but rather the moral foundation for practical-political control over technology. The urgency to ground the principle of responsibility is not theoretical but practical; only a principle free from suspicion of arbitrariness can legitimate control over the political and economic forces that fuel utopian ambitions (Jonas, 1984, pp. 25–26).

RESPONSIBILITY IN PRACTICE

One who has followed Jonas's argument is likely to be disappointed that the result of these herculean labors is a mere responsibility for the continued existence of responsible beings. This responsibility requires us to keep the capacity for responsibility alive but does not tell us how to exercise responsibility in less critical but still urgent conditions where the capacity itself is not threatened. It does not tell us specifically what kinds of biomedical interventions are morally unacceptable. Are we left with an apocalyptic ethic that applies only to the limit cases of our current biomedical technology?[18]

The principle of responsibility itself is directly relevant to at least one concrete moral issue, namely human experimentation. In other cases it is indirectly relevant, though as I show below the kind of purposiveness humans are responsible for must be rendered more determinate in order for its relevance to appear. The key to Jonas's treatment of human experimentation is his recognition that biomedical progress is gratuitous and participation in it therefore nonobligatory. "The destination of research is essentially melioristic. . . . Unless the present state is intolerable, the melioristic goal is in a sense gratuitous . . ." (Jonas, 1974, p. 117). At the same time, however, progress involves a certain nobility which must also be taken into consideration. "Both the nobility and the gratuitousness must influence the manner in which self-sacrifice for it is elicited, and even its free offer accepted" (Jonas, 1974, p. 118). The result is that except in those very rare cases when disaster must be averted, the motivation and norm for participation in nontherapeutic research must be found in "the sublime solitude of dedication and ultimate commitment, . . . the sphere of the holy" (Jonas, 1974, p. 119).

But why this stringent criterion? Why require more than the subject's consent? Because for Jonas the chief ethical problem with making a person a subject of nontherapeutic research "is not so much that we make him thereby a means (which happens in social contexts of all kinds), as that we make him a thing. . . . His being is reduced to that of a mere token or 'sample'" (Jonas, 1974, p. 107). This wrong cannot be overcome by self-determination. "Mere consent . . . does not right this reification" (Jonas, 1974, p. 108). Jonas obviously presupposes a strong view of humans as ends, one for which not self-determination but ontological status is the issue. But his essay simply posits that view; it never elaborates it or justifies it. Although the essay precedes Jonas's development of the principle of responsibility, it requires something like the unconditional duty to preserve and not violate the conditions of responsibility. The argument stands, in other words, only if nontherapeutic experimentation potentially constitutes a violation of the duty to maintain purposiveness as a good in itself, a good that is threatened, however momentarily, by becoming a research subject. If one recalls that, as the ought-to-be of a good in itself, such a duty stands above both researcher and subject, then it is clear why consent cannot right this wrong. Only by bringing the fullness of purposiveness itself into the experimental process is reduction to thinghood avoided. For this reason, the criterion for eliciting and accepting participation is for Jonas (purposive) identification with the project iself, not consent.[19]

If I am right that the principle of responsibility supplies the missing ground for Jonas's stringent requirement, I must admit that Jonas's next move is puzzling. Recognizing that such a criterion would restrict participation to scientists and a handful of other educated elites who alone would be capable of genuinely identifying with the project, thus making it impossible to obtain sufficient numbers for a significant sample, Jonas permits a rule of descending order from these ideal conditions of motivation. In practice, this means that identification is a matter of degree and that recruitment of subjects proceeds according to their approximation to full identification. But on what grounds can Jonas allow such a declension? If reduction to thinghood is intrinsically wrong unless there is genuine identification, and if progress is optional, how can such a wrong be permitted for the sake of what is optional? The declension seems to be justifiable only in the case of a disaster, where progress is not optional and such a declension seems to be one reasonable way of eliciting participation. However, Jonas does indicate that only a "residue of identification" is necessary. This yields a general principle that the less of a residue there is, the closer the cause of the experimental project must be to the limit case of the disaster, which would seem to validate the declension (Jonas, 1974, p. 129). But if only a "residue of identification" is necessary, how does this residue differ from mere consent, which Jonas has already told us is necessary but not sufficient? Jonas seems to be left with the alternatives of a de facto moratorium on nontherapeutic experimentation in nondisaster situations or recognition of a spectrum of risks and benefits in which full identification would be merely an ideal case.

Up to now Jonas's concern has been the threats various forms of technology pose to the very existence of humans as responsible beings. But technology potentially affects human nature in profound ways even when it does not put the existence of humans as responsible beings at stake. There is therefore a need for a more substantive conception of the purposiveness humans are responsible for. Can Jonas supply such a conception? It is reasonable to seek one in his earlier conception of organism. We saw above that for Jonas metabolism is the basis for a complex ontology of organism. We noted there the polarity of being and not-being: unlike inorganic matter, organisms never possess their being in a persistent state but realize it by continuous self-performance. In contrast to inorganic matter, organisms therefore possess a certain freedom with regard to their own matter yet for the same reason (namely its transcendence, through self-performance, of the matter of which it consists) are utterly dependent on their environment for exchange of matter—an environment that may deny them what they need. Hence in addition to the polarity of being and not-being inherent in the being of the organism as self-performance, Jonas recognizes polarities of freedom and necessity and self and world (Jonas, 1966, pp. 83–86; 1974, pp. 194–196). As organisms become more complex their existence is more tenuous, the distinction between self and world departing further and further from the "neutral assuredness of existence" that follows from the complete identity of the inorganic with its matter, and requiring progressively more complex faculties (from metabolism to motility and perception to image making) to secure existence.

Two important points follow from this increasing complexity of life. First, while the freedom of the organism vis-à-vis its environment increases as one ascends the scale, the venture of life becomes increasingly perilous. This indicates that life strives for something more than assuredness of existence; Jonas agrees with Nietzsche against Darwin that the survival standard is inadequate: "If mere assurance of permanence were the point that mattered, life should not have started out in the first place." Rather, "means" of survival such as greater motility, emotional capacity or refinement of vision become qualities to be preserved and thus part of an ever more complex end. "It is one of the paradoxes of life that it employs means which modify the end and themselves become part of it" (Jonas, 1966, p. 106). But life pays a survival price for its increasing richness, and is thus "an experiment with mounting stakes and risks which in the fateful freedom of man may end in disaster as well as success" (Jonas, 1966, p. x). Second, as the inwardness implied in the concern for being develops, a progressively more concentrated and focused subject is set off against a progressively more disinct world. Motility and emotion play an important role here, but with the development of sight the world can be held at a distance from engagement with it. When this capacity is granted primacy, it makes possible the world as pure extension realized by a subject who is thus able to stand over against it (Jonas, 1966, pp. 146–54). Further up the scale, the capacity for making images makes possible an even greater progression of objectification: from the remaking of things, to the making of new things, and finally to the remaking of the maker (Jonas, 1966, 172–173, 185–186). Hence the capacities for sight and image making supply the ontological grounds for the attitudes and practices of the Baconian subject. But clearly the capacities of sight and image making do not necessarily produce the modern subject. What then accounts for his existence? It seems that the condition for such a subject is his forgetfulness of the earlier stages of organic being on which his objectifying capacities rest. Under the spell of his powers of objectification, technological man is in danger of forgetting the originary imbeddedness in the world that makes these capacities possible. The tension of freedom and peril reaches its highest pitch as the freedom inherent in modern technology courts the peril of the destruction of human freedom itself.

Does this ontology of the organism yield a more substantive conception of the human? While for Aristotle the good is what completes or perfects a being, the nature of the organism as continuous self-performance of its being indicates that its telos can not be a state of completion. Instead, "the *telos* of the organic individual, the teleology of individuality as such, is the acting out of the very tension of the polarities that constitute its being, and thus the *process* of its existence as such" (Jonas, 1974, p. 197). What is normatively human in this broader sense, then, is the acting out of the tensions of the polarities, and one violates the normatively human by acting out one pole to the exclusion or denigration of the other. Is this sufficient to resolve bioethical issues in which the existence of humans as purposive is not immediately at stake? It seems at least to provide a negative criterion. I will now show how for Jonas what I will call the forgetfulness of organic being stands behind all of the proposals for biomedical engineering. As he sees them, they all in one way or another constitute a Baconian effort to exalt one side of the polarities that constitute our being over the other and to deny that other. The Baconian project itself is based on the effort to eliminate necessity in favor of freedom or, to use Pascal's famous image, to deny that humanity is a reed as well as a thinker. Apart from its threat to the capacity for responsibility, it is the flattening out of these polarities, the elimination of the ambiguities that constitute human existence, that Jonas fears most from modern technology (cf. Jonas, 1984, pp. 200–201).

The application of this conception of the human to a concrete bioethical issue is perhaps most clear in the case Jonas makes for mortality as both a burden and a blessing. Mortality is a burden insofar as we organic beings must wrest our being from the continuous threat of nonbeing. But it is a blessing insofar as our wresting is the very condition for any affirmation of being at all, so that "mortality is the narrow gate through which alone *value*—the addressee of a yes—could enter the otherwise indifferent universe" (Jonas, 1992, p. 36). Consequently, the effort to forestall aging or even mortality itself, if it ever comes to that, is a fundamental denial of what makes us human. But metabolism alone does not clinch the argument. The process of life, Jonas (following Hannah Arendt) argues, requires mortality as the counterpart of the natality that alone can supply the novelty and creativity that enrich human life and express freedom (Jonas, 1992, p. 39). Freedom itself, it seems, is imperiled when it ignores necessity.

In the case of other ethical issues, the argument is more complex and the role of this conception of the human is less direct. But I believe it is still determinative, as I will now show in Jonas's discussions of eugenics and genetic engineering. In regard to negative eugenics, Jonas argues for the legitimacy of restoring in the population as a whole the balance of nature interfered with in order to save individuals from their genetic fates through biomedical intervention. Prevention of reproduction by those enabled by medicine to live long enough to reproduce is therefore a legitimate goal, though Jonas is careful to note that the means of restraint (which range from persuasion to sterilization) raise moral problems of their own. The argument has a consequentialist flavor: geneticists at the time Jonas wrote were predicting that the ability of medicine to keep such persons alive to reproduce would eventually result in a severely debilitated gene pool. But Jonas's major worry is that our concern about the gene pool will lead us toward overly ambitious eugenic goals that go beyond maintaining at the population level the genetic status quo that we have altered for the sake of individuals. Here his argument is mixed. He first appeals to a normative status for nature itself, which more ambitious eugenic concerns could violate, and hints at our lack of criteria or standards for determining what is normal and what is pathogenic. "Thus the remedial zeal can easily . . . widen the concept 'pathogenic' to include the 'undesirable' in more arbitrary senses and then forfeit the sanction of nature" beyond compensation for what natural selection would have done without our medical intervention for the sake of individuals. "The same goes for the temptation to extend the control . . . to . . . recessive carriers." However, there are also consequentialist concerns with these efforts to eliminate "bad genes" from the population: any effort to eliminate undesirable genes from the gene pool altogether threatens the biological necessity of a varied gene pool and encounters our ignorance about the role apparently useless genes may play in human adaptability. In any case, the goal of merely maintaining a balance at the population level that medicine has interfered with at the individual level avoids all of these problems posed by more ambitious eugenic proposals (Jonas, 1974, pp. 146–148).[20]

Jonas's arguments against positive eugenics are similar to those against ambitious forms of negative eugenics. Once again there are appeals to the normative status of nature and to our lack of criteria and standards for intervention. Since positive eugenics aims at a qualitative improvement over nature, it can not claim the sanction of nature. Just as the more ambitious proposals for negative eugenics raise questions about what constitutes "pathogenic," so positive eugenics raises questions about what criteria or standards should determine what counts as "improvement." Finally, there is the consequentialist argument: our efforts to standardize certain desired human traits once again threatens the variety of the gene pool and encounters our ignorance about this variety (Jonas, 1974, pp. 151–153).

Genetic engineering raises the same problems about standards or criteria and, in the case of germ-line interventions, some of the same questions about the ultimate consequences for the gene pool as a whole. Despite insisting on the lack of standards or criteria, Jonas does not hesitate to designate many ends of genetic engineering, such as most uses of human growth hormones, to be frivolous (Jonas, 1985, pp. 495–496). But granting that we can without a more substantive view of the good distinguish serious and frivolous interventions, what about serious uses of germ-line gene therapy for debilitating diseases? Here Jonas appeals almost exclusively to consequences: the irreversibility of germ-line interventions, the range of their effects, the impossibility of drawing a line in practice between therapy and enhancement of traits or prohibiting the outright invention of new human forms that violate the ontological status of human nature (Jonas, 1985, pp. 502–504).

Leaving aside the wrongness of certain means of achieving these ends (e.g., experimentation on the unborn, who can not identify with the aims), Jonas appears to approach all three of these issues with three kinds of consideration in mind: the consequences of our actions, which in a technological era are largely unknown and in many cases irreversible, the integrity of nature, and the lack of a conception of the human capable of providing criteria or standards for which improvements we ought to aim at. But it is not clear whether the three considerations are compatible. If the integrity of nature serves as an absolute norm rendering certain interventions impermissible, why does Jonas appeal to consequences? Conversely, if consequences are decisive, what role does the integrity of nature play in the argument? And in either case, what is the role of our lack of a fully substantive conception of the human? I suggest that the argument is something like the following. Nature itself endorses no fully substantive conception of the human as normative but only the process of acting out the polarities. All of our conceptions for the improvement of humanity over what nature accomplishes on its own are therefore necessarily arbitrary and ephemeral. Lacking the sanction of nature, in the absence of an extreme emergency they are nonobligatory. Granted this, consequential considerations carry the day: since improvements are by definition melioristic rather than necessary, the threats of severe consequences should prevent us from carrying them out at all. The principle is that aside from supreme emergencies the burden of proof is on intervention to show that it can do better than nature has done. Given our arbitrary con-

ceptions of the human and the magnitude of the potential consequences under conditions of modern technology, it is a heavy burden
indeed. In short, the key principle is not the integrity of the course of
nature as an absolute value but rather the absence of wisdom, which
renders our thick conceptions of human nature arbitrary and
ephemeral. "Imagine it, and ask yourself whether it is good and
wise . . . to meddle for ephemeral-hedonistic reasons with the ways of
nature, who here has set her own times by the long trial of evolution"
(Jonas, 1985, p. 496). The whimsicality and constant shifting of our
goals—in contrast to the range and endurance of their effects and to the
gradual and time-tested way in which nature establishes ends—coun-
sels restraint. Human nature, normatively considered, just *is* the living
out of the polarities that constitute it, and therefore is always in process
but never still to be realized. To seek to realize our own fleeting conceptions is to terminate the process in favor of one arbitrary distortion
of it. Put in religious terms, "we simply must not try to fixate man in
any image of our own definition and thereby cut off the as yet unre-
vealed promises of the image of God" (Jonas, 1974, p. 181).

In sum, to be responsible for responsibility is, concretely, to preserve in the face of technology the human project of acting out the polarities. Humanity already is, and is not still to be realized through our
utopian ambitions.

EVALUATION

The legacy of the Baconian-Cartesian revolt against classical conceptions of human nature is for Jonas the utopian premise that humanity is yet to realized, the nihilistic premise that there is no objective
good that can ground a normative conception of the human, and the
practical premise that whatever human destiny is, it is to be achieved by
technological control of nature. In order to overcome this nihilistic
utopianism without returning to the classical position, Jonas must show
how something subject to our power is nevertheless an objective good
that makes claims against that power, and that the material nature (artificiality) and formal dynamics (automatic progress) of modern technology therefore involve the Baconian subject in a dialectic that threatens to destroy that objective good. His argument follows accordingly:
the continued existence of a humanity capable of exercising responsibility is an unconditional duty imposed on human power; biomedical
practices and interventions that threaten responsibility are therefore
morally unacceptable.

Aside from the interpretation of technological utopianism that requires it, how sound is the argument itself? We have seen that it depends on two premises: a formal premise regarding the relation between good and ought and a material premise consisting of claims regarding the objectivity of purposiveness, its intrinsic goodness, and the primacy of responsibility for human purposiveness. I will take them in reverse order, concentrating on the final two claims. Jonas's formulation of the primacy of responsibility for other humans takes the reversibility of responsibility for other humans—that the object of my responsibility is also a subject who is responsible just as I am—as a conclusive reason for the primacy of this kind of responsibility. However, the shareability of responsibility for human beings (I am responsible for others who are also responsible, and thus am uniquely able to make their purposiveness my own purpose) is not an argument for its primacy. Nevertheless it is possible to construct a stronger argument from Jonas's own premises. The key premise is that a good-in-itself becomes a duty for an agent when it depends on that agent to bring it about. Human beings alone possess the capacity to be responsible for the purposiveness of others, that is, to make the purposiveness of another their own purpose. Moreover, of human beings alone is it true that their purposiveness can be brought about only if other human beings are in fact responsible for it; for all other beings purposiveness realizes itself without anyone's becoming responsible for it. But if (1) human beings alone *can* be responsible, and (2) the intrinsic good of purposiveness in the case of human beings, and them alone, can be brought about only if human beings *are* responsible for it, it follows that human beings *must* be responsible for their fellow human beings in a way that they are not responsible for other beings, whose purposiveness does not depend on human responsibility for its actualization. The actualization of the intrinsic right-to-be of human purposiveness requires that humans take responsibility for it in a way that is not necessary for the actualization of purposiveness in any other being. Interestingly, this argument does not entail the claim that responsibility, the form purposiveness takes in human beings, is superior to the purposiveness of other beings, or even that the primacy of responsibility to human beings implies a valuation of humans above other beings—although Jonas believes his argument does require this (Jonas, 1984, pp. 233–234, n. 3).[21]

Next is the moral-ontological argument for the intrinsic goodness and ought-to-be-ness of purposiveness itself. Jonas must show that there is not only a negative duty not to put humanity itself at risk for melioristic gains but a positive duty for the continuation of human beings as responsible agents. The argument works only if purposiveness as the capacity for value difference is necessarily an intrinsic good absolutely superior to the absence of value difference. But Jonas's argument does not support this claim. Because the intrinsic goodness of purposiveness is not logically or transcendentally entailed in its objectivity, the move from being to goodness is not a necessary move. One could say without logical or performative self-contradiction, "In positing itself against nonbeing, being affirms value difference over value indifference, but I am indifferent toward this affirmation," or even, "I am not sure whether value difference is a good thing or not." Jonas recognizes this and therefore tries to make the connection between being and goodness in the two ways noted above: a cognitivist appeal to an intuition of the intrinsic goodness of purposiveness over nonpurposiveness and a noncognitivist appeal to a metaphysical choice for the former over the latter. But without a necessary link between purposiveness and goodness, the argument fails as a moral-ontological argument; the concept of purposive being does not require its existence as an ought. This does not mean that there are no possible connections between being and goodness or is and ought, but only that any such connections are not necessary in the sense Jonas's moral-ontological argument requires. But if they are not necessary in this sense and if his argument depends on their being such, Jonas has not succeeded in refuting the nihilistic utopians.

Having challenged the heart of Jonas's project I can be brief with the remaining two points, both of which require and merit a lengthy discussion. First, Jonas's shift from the extrapolation from my own purposiveness to that of organic life in general to the *via negativa* that vindicates subjective testimony by refuting metaphysical arguments that deny such testimony is a philosophical gain but Jonas still conducts the debate in the discourse of classical mechanics.[22] Second, that the intrinsic goodness of something not yet existing entails a positive ought to realize it is not self-evident and is almost certainly not true apart from additional premises, though the intrinsic goodness of something already existing is a prima facie reason for not destroying it or for maintaining it in existence.

The major problem is that Jonas's argument fails as a rationalistic argument to mediate between the description of nature in terms of purposiveness, the intuition of and choice for purposiveness as an intrinsic good, and the realization of purposiveness as a duty. (In the following chapter I examine James Gustafson's more explicit attempt at a similar mediation between a description of nature and its normative significance, and his use of theological claims to accomplish it.) Jonas was aware of the limitations of his argument as a rationalistic argument, even wondering whether the duty to the future existence of humanity is not altogether beyond the scope of reason (Jonas, 1982, p. 209). He repeatedly warned his readers that his arguments could not provide the finality that the claims of religious ethics have for believers, thus devaluing his own rationalistic currency even as he issued it (Jonas, 1982, pp. 208–209; 1984, pp. 23, 45). Yet he continued to try to establish this duty on philosophical grounds because these grounds alone would give the principle the public authority needed to enact it in the political realm (Jonas, 1984, pp. 25–26).

But if the student of Heidegger (and of classical Jewish philosophy) was careful to distinguish reflection on revealed truths from philosophical inquiry, the student of Rudolf Bultmann could not resist repeated attempts to formulate his major points in theological terms. One of these attempts was a Lurianic-Hegelian speculative myth according to which God renounces his own being in order for the world to be and thereby entrusts his own destiny to that of the world, to be recovered in its becoming. Eventually in the course of things the divine destiny passes into human trust, where human freedom renders it precarious and human deeds—good and evil—therefore have transcendent importance (Jonas, 1966, pp. 275–281). While designed to address problems of immortality and evil the myth also makes humans responsible for the very image of God, which their deeds could destroy. Less systematically, Jonas also regularly applied the language of Genesis 1— reverence for creation as intrinsically good, respect for humanity in the image of God, human dominion over a good creation as stewardship— in predictable ways to his concerns with modern technology. Given this immersion in the Judaic tradition one wonders whether the importance Jonas attached to the duty to continue the existence of humanity ultimately reflects (and disguises) in rational and universalistic terms the importance of the mitzvah of procreation in Judaism.[23] If so, Jonas's failure to supply a rational ground for this commandment and thereby demonstrate its validity for humanity as a whole is further evidence that reason alone cannot compensate for what is lost with the abandonment of religious traditions.

So much for the argument for responsibility. We must now consider Jonas's claims that humanity is always already realized in the polarities that constitute the human organism and that, in cases where the very existence of humanity is not at stake, the absence of an objectively valid, more substantive conception of the human means that the dangers and uncertainty attending the consequences of our actions require us to reject all efforts to go beyond what nature accomplishes in the polarities. There are two problems with Jonas's conception of the human as the living out of these polarities. The first problem is that Jonas claims to arrive at the polarities by a phenomenological analysis but occasionally uses the polarities as a theoretical framework. In part because of this, the polarities often reintroduce the very dualism Jonas thought he had transcended.[24] The second problem is that the redescription of teleology as the living out of the polarities is unable to resolve with the authority Jonas seeks the bioethical issues for which it seems best suited, namely those in which the future existence of humanity as responsible is not immediately at stake. The reason is that simply to live out the polarities themselves is to indicate nothing about *how* we should balance freedom and necessity, only *that* we must do so. In the case of somatic cell engineering, for example, this alone is not sufficient to distinguish between "frivolous" (enhancement) and "serious" (therapy) uses. Moreover, the argument from the absence of a more substantive teleology can work against Jonas as well as for him. The convinced Baconian could argue that by designating all improvements as melioristic and thus purely optional, Jonas has already decided in favor of necessity against freedom. If freedom is genuinely part of human nature, it is a mistake to designate all efforts to lift humanity beyond the grip of necessity as melioristic and to ignore the consequences of failing to give freedom its due. Jonas has no effective reply to this argument because without a more substantive view of the good he cannot tell us how to balance freedom and necessity.

In short, Jonas's argument continues and thereby reaffirms the discourse of the modern subject. By accepting the terms of this discourse, Jonas can only develop his responsible subject as a corrective reversal of the Baconian subject, not as a genuine alternative to it. If the Baconian project emphasized freedom at the expense of necessity, Jonas will emphasize the latter, pointing out the ignorance and foolishness of our arbitary freedom and urging us therefore to let nature (necessity) run its own course in the case of eugenics and gene therapy. The result is that rather than transcending the modern subject, Jonas can succeed, if at all, only in redressing an imbalance in the usual conceptions of the latter. The irony is that while Jonas and others who share his views are often perceived as being antitechnological, they are in many respects as modern as the Baconians they criticize.

This leaves us with the final question, which determines the relevance of everything else, namely Jonas's interpretation of technology. Ironically, at the very point at which he seeks to break with Bacon, Jonas is deeply entangled in the Baconian framework. First, he constructs technology entirely on an opposition between artificial and natural. Aside from the fact that an inextricable intertwining of "natural" and "artificial" began with the development of the human brain, this opposition valorizes the Baconian narrative of technology as the triumph of freedom (artificiality) over necessity (nature). That this triumph eventually turns Baconian freedom against itself in the form of a new necessity does not itself undermine the Baconian subject; the dialectic occurs wholly within the economy of this subject. Concretely, this means that the triumph of artificiality that dialectically coils back on the subject will exhibit the same totality that characterized the subject's own control. Hence for Jonas any initial step in the direction of genetic or neurological engineering inevitably heralds total technological control of life and the end of purposiveness altogether. Technological control itself, that is, takes the form of a Baconian totalizing subject while the development from mechanics to molecular biology, and the formal dynamics of progress that underwrites it, is the metanarrative of its inevitable triumph.

Given this interpretation, Jonas ultimately must understand responsibility itself in quasi-Baconian terms as gaining power over power or regaining control over what now threatens to control us (Jonas, 1979, p. 41; 1984, p. 142). In other words, the responsible subject, however defined by its care for what has come under the guilt of its power, is still essentially a modern subject who must gain control over technology in order to remain a subject at all (or at least a responsible one). It is difficult to overemphasize the importance this effort to gain control has for Jonas. First, it determines the need for rationally compelling arguments, since only the latter can legitimize the political power that will be needed to control technology. Second, it determines Jonas's conception of politics. Political theory for him reduces to the question of which system, Marxism or capitalism, is more likely to gain control over the dynamics of technology. Convinced that the technological threat to the human is inevitable but aware that its urgency is not apparent to the public, Jonas recommends the Platonic noble lie as a strategy to ensure that the wisdom of the philosopher will prevail in the cave of politics, and even advocates surreptitious uses of technology itself to the same end (Jonas, 1979, p. 42; 1984, pp. 142–157).

In contrast to Jonas I doubt that it is possible to gain control over technology, partly because I believe that technology has already dispersed the Baconian subject into complex networks of power, and that the danger of the Baconian project and its utopianism is not that it will destroy our purposiveness but that it will form us in certain ways as certain kinds of subjects. I therefore argue in the final chapter that the task is not to gain control over technology but to be guided by a process of moral formation that is capable of both resisting its diffuse power and assimilating it into a moral project. This presupposes a subject who no longer pretends to master nature or even to master the technology that masters nature.

Despite these shortcomings, our trek through Jonas's complex arguments has been worthwhile. He has showed us how fragile is the ethic that underlies the Baconian project: how easily the technology sought in fulfilment of ethical purposes transforms these very purposes into a nihilistic form of utopianism. As a result, the picture I presented in chapter one has gained a sharper focus, richer detail, and more depth. More constructively, Jonas has drawn our attention to the body as a focus for an alternative bioethic, even if he could not finally escape the modern framework for understanding the body. Finally, if Jonas himself did not deconstruct the Baconian subject, his dialectical understanding of that subject's power prepares us to understand how technology can be simultaneously the greatest exercise of human power and the greatest form of power over humanity.

CHAPTER 4

Medicine and the Ethics of Vocation

In 1984 James Gustafson explained to his readers the reason for the attention he had given to ethical issues in the biological sciences for much of his career.

> Over the past twenty years I have, in a lay person's way, attempted to grasp the main lines of genetic and neurological research because I believe that in biology these have the widest implications for future human participation. Man, in my judgment, will come closer to being the ultimate orderer of life through the uses of these investigations than through the matters that preoccupy so much of the attention in clinical medical ethics. Of course in practice it will not be "man" but those persons and institutions that have the power to control the use of such investigations. (Gustafson, 1984, pp. 281–282, n. 2)

It may appear strange to introduce Gustafson's work with a footnote buried deep in the second volume of his magnum opus, *Ethics from a Theocentric Perspective* (hereafter ETP). But to understand Gustafson's work in bioethics and even in theological ethics more generally one must understand why the arena of biomedical research serves as an appropriate point of entry and how the issues it raises strike at the very core of his agenda. For Gustafson, I will argue, more than any other figure in theological ethics understands both the achievements and the limitations of the Baconian project of relieving the human condition, and is deeply attuned to both the promises and the perils that accompany human efforts to displace God as the ultimate orderer of life.

AN ETHIC OF VOCATION

For Gustafson the chief question of ethics is "What is God enabling and requiring us to be and do?" The answer falls within a familiar tradition: the classical Protestant ethics of vocation with its moral valuation of ordinary life as Taylor has described it. Gustafson's subtle and complex relation to this tradition determines his fundamental metaphor for human being and acting (human beings as "participants" in natural and social processes), as well as the fundamental problem ethics addresses, the nature of moral reasoning, and the selection of topics for moral consideration. Or so I will argue. At this stage it is necessary to make two preliminary points. First, Gustafson's ethic of vocation is best seen as a provisional answer to the chief question that has occupied him for a quarter century: What is the normatively human? How do we determine it, and how are our descriptions related to our normative conclusions? That the answer to this question is connected with the idea of vocation is clear from an early investigation where Gustafson ends an analytical treatment of the issue of the normatively human with a constructive conclusion: "My strong hunch is that to be human is to have a vocation, a calling; that it is to become what we now are not; that it calls for a surpassing of what we are; that apart from a telos, a vision of what man can and ought to do, we will flounder and decay" (Gustafson, 1974, p. 244).

The emphasis on transcending the present reflects concerns of both Protestant and Catholic theologians at the time to overcome static and essentialist anthropologies. But it also gives a clue to the nature of vocation. This is the second point. Gustafson's work exhibits the chief characteristics of the Calvinist version of the ethic of vocation, with its emphasis on discipline, intense activity in the world, the sins of pride and sloth, and the conformity or ordering of the world to the will of God (cf. Troeltsch, 1931, pp. 602–612).[1] In a summary of the theocentric orientation that governs ETP Gustafson put the point succinctly in language that recalls John Calvin. "Piety . . . demands . . . the disciplining of life, the ordering of human communities, the relating of human activity and culture to the natural world in ways that recognize both human finitude and the human defect, and recognizes that life must be conformed to that ordering activity of God which we cannot fully know" (Gustafson, 1982b, p. 91). These characteristics also include moral and theological justification of human use of and control over the natural world for the improvement of ordinary life and confers moral significance on the development and exercise of technical skills; Gustafson drinks from the same well as Bacon (Gustafson, 1981, pp. 3–7; 1983, p. 496). But Gustafson has also faced the dangers of the Baconian project in an era when the capacity to relieve the human condition harbors potentially destructive consequences for human beings and for nature. Hence the most distinguishing feature of Gustafson's ethics, and the feature that elicits the most moral passion in Gustafson and in his critics, is his powerful sense of the limits to and dangers of the Baconian agenda. These limits and dangers strongly qualify the moral approval given to efforts to use and control nature and introduce great complexity into the notion of vocation.

Working from within the ethic of vocation, then, the human capacity to intervene into nature, including human nature, and the limitations and consequences of this capacity constitute the problem that Gustafson's ethics seeks to address. Gustafson begins ETP with an interpretation of the circumstances that warrant the particular type of theological ethics he offers. First in this interpretation is a description of human culture as a progression of control over fate. "One of the persistent characteristics of human beings since the dawn of consciousness is that our species extends the range of its domination over forces and powers deemed at first beyond its control, for the sake of greater security to individuals and communities" (Gustafson, 1981, pp. 3–4). Other purposes besides security are mentioned: the relief of suffering, the betterment of health, the enrichment of human experience. It is worthwhile to pause here since Gustafson has identified a characteristic of human nature and activity that occupies a determining role in his ethics. Human nature and activity are not described in Aristotelian terms (the pursuit of the virtues in the life of the polis), Augustinian terms (the orientation of the will to God), Hobbesian terms (the pursuit of individual happiness) or Kantian terms (the governance of life by autonomous reason). Rather it is essentially Baconian: technological man or, to add to H. Richard Niebuhr's well known three types, "man the intervener" (cf. Niebuhr, 1963). The most significant feature of human beings is their remarkable capacity to intervene into nature, including human nature.

As I show below, this has far-reaching implications for nature itself, but here I wish only to indicate its importance for how Gustafson construes the task of ethics. Gustafson quickly follows up his recognition of human intervention with a strong conviction about the limitations of intervention. His account of these limitations includes several features. The first is that our interventions seldom complete their purpose of overcoming fate or necessity. Insecurity, for example, is not eliminated but evoked by new objects (Gustafson, 1984, p. 5). Beneficial and deleterious consequences of human interventions inexorably occur together. Human beings overcome many limits of necessity but not "the most fundamental limitations of constituting a biological species, of being dependent upon and interdependent with other persons, institutions, and culture, and the natural environment around us" (Gustafson, 1984, p. 14). Gustafson sometimes criticizes certain biomedical practices (e.g., efforts to extend biological life indefinitely) for their presumptuous denials of these constitutional limitations. The second is that human knowledge of and control over the effects of their interventions is limited. The result is that interventions always involve risks. Here Gustafson largely concurs with Hans Jonas's account of the altered character of human action considered in chapter three. "The time and space scopes of the consequences of human interventions into nature and into social processes have expanded without the commensurate increase in humility that is proper, given the continuing remarkable limitations of foreknowledge of long-range consequences and of the capacity to control them" (Gustafson, 1982b, p. 84). Like Jonas, Gustafson is deeply concerned about the disparity between the range and cumulative nature of the effects of human interventions made possible by technology and the lack of knowledge of or control over those effects. The expanded scope of human action requires both consideration of a much wider range of consequences than is often considered and refraining from (or at least proceeding with extreme caution in) interventions for which these consequences are unknown or unexplored. An example is biomedical research designed to slow or arrest aging processes (Gustafson, 1984, pp. 264–265, n. 9).

While these features point to human finitude that is never overcome, the last comment indicates human failure or fault (Gustafson avoids the language of sin in his later work as assiduously as he avoids personal language for God) in the two forms emphasized most by Calvin, namely pride and sloth. Pride refers to the human pretensions of mastery over nature and the potential dangers this courts. But it may also refer to tendencies to exercise power over others and to put individual self-fulfillment or one's professional community ahead of one's obligations to others (Gustafson, 1975b, pp. 71–72). Sloth refers to the human tendency to rest satisfied with conditions as they now are and to resist or ignore new possibilities in the orderings of nature and history.

It is clear that recognition of most of these limitations backs concerns for restraining human interventions. Indeed Gustafson's chief concern is to temper the ambitions of the Baconian project. But as the concern with sloth indicates, Gustafson has no interest in overturning that project altogether. Human beings are accountable for the possibilities they ignore as well as for the limitations they deny. The attention to new possibilities of achieving well-being or avoiding harmful states of affairs for humans and others means that traditional principles and orderings of values may be altered—a claim by which Gustafson sharply distinguishes himself from Paul Ramsey (Gustafson, 1975b, pp. 37–38, 44–45). But in addition to their moral significance, these limitations also carry great theological significance. Three times in the discussion that opens ETP volume 1, Gustafson points to limitations as a vivid reminder that despite our uncertainty about whether God exists, we can be certain that human beings are not God (Gustafson, 1981, pp. 9, 13, 16).

Human beings, then, are interveners, but limited ones. Or in Gustafson's own elegant words summarizing various human interventions,

> These illustrations indicate that modern societies and cultures, as well as individual persons, are gifted with capacities and possibilities that are naturally and properly exercised to increase control over what were formerly contingencies, accidents, matters subject to fate or to the irrational determination of the gods—to necessity, however it has been symbolized. They also indicate that to be human, in spite of the vastness of human achievements, is to be limited. (Gustafson, 1981, p. 8)[2]

Three points follow. First, while Gustafson's entire ethics is an ethics of vocation, the potential for unprecedented destruction of human beings and nature that comes in the wake of the expanded range of human action introduces a complication into the classical Calvinist idea of vocation. While a Bacon or a John Locke, for example, could rest assured that the purposes of God for humans and nature are fulfilled by reducing nature to human control and using it "for the Support and Comfort of their being" (Locke, 1960, p. 328), Gustafson can entertain no such confidence knowing that nature does not guarantee such support and comfort and that the technological efforts to force it to do so can be catastrophic. While for Bacon and the Puritans there was no conflict between controlling nature for human benefit and the glory of God, we know that if we continue to exercise our powers of intervention with human benefit and well-being as the only criteria and to ignore the limits of our knowledge and control, we will imperil human beings and the rest of nature. Hence for Gustafson the preservation and enhancement of ordinary human life by the agency of medicine or any other vocation must also reckon with the risks and costs and limits of controlling nature itself toward this end.

Second, Gustafson's emphasis on vocation or participation determines the types of moral issues he raises and the concepts and methods of moral reasoning he employs. If the morally significant characteristic of humans is their capacity to intervene into natural processes, a different set of questions will come to the fore than if the chief characteristic is faithfulness to a covenant or to a norm or ideal, or cultivation of virtues. This is clear from some of the questions Gustafson identifies early on in ETP and which he pursues throughout: What values ought to be pursued in our interventions? What purposes ought to govern the human drive toward mastery over the forces to which they remain subject? At what point do humans deny or try to overcome natural finitude? What are the proper responses to the recognition of finitude and fault? Most important, do our capacities for control justify the inference that all other things exist for human benefit? (Gustafson, 1981, p. 15).

Third, we now have a provisional answer to the question of why biomedical research is Gustafson's point of entry into bioethics. This kind of research marks the most crucial points of intervention into natural processes, and thus the points where human vocation or participation is most effectually exercised. Here is where values, purposes, and limits must be determined, and where the greatest possibilities but also the greatest threats for human beings and nature are located. Biomedical research provides an ideal locus for exploring and testing an ethics that seeks to come to terms with Bacon.

One final point will complete this sketch of Gustafson's view of vocation. Ordinary human inclinations and capacities are morally significant for Gustafson, and their formation and development in a moral community is a moral and religious duty: to participate "requires attention to our capacities to be participants, to sustain and develop the necessary conditions to function in our roles." Gustafson agrees with Kant (and by implication with Luther) that the cultivation of skills and moral virtues is other-regarding; duties to self are a form of duties to others. But Gustafson expands this to include not only duties but aspirations, and not only for individual humans but for "the species, society, culture, and even nature" (Gustafson, 1984, p. 285). However, vocation is not entirely other-regarding. From early on Gustafson recognized that human life has both intrinsic and instrumental value (Gustafson, 1971, pp. 147–148), and when he raises the question of whether human life ever loses its value he consistently refers to its value for self as well as for the community (Gustafson, 1984, pp. 214–215).[3] What the primacy of vocation does rule out is the priority of one's own moral perfection over one's responsibilities for the well-being of others.[4]

I have now presented the basic shape and direction of the moral life in Gustafson's theological ethics. It consists of "a sense of calling, a vocation, that is both a responsibility and an opportunity, to participate in the developing of life in the world toward those ends that we can judge to be morally worthy" (Gustafson, 1984, p. 42). But equally and perhaps even more important is the "prophetic thrust which reminds us that only God is God" (Gustafson, 1984, p. 40) that Gustafson finds in Karl Barth's theology. This conviction hovers over the sense of human limitation and ultimately ensures that vocation involves being "a participant in and a caretaker of a world that is given by God" (Gustafson, 1984, pp. 40–41). These convictions, along with his ecclesiology (which I do not discuss), constitute the Protestant side of Gustafson's theocentric ethics. It is now time to turn to a side that combines Protestant and Catholic features.

THE SOURCES OF MORAL INSIGHT

If the provisional answer to the question of the normatively human is the notion of vocation, the next question for genetic, neurological and other medical research is whether there is a more substantive answer; an idea of the normatively human that would serve as a criterion for responsible intervention. The task of theological ethics more generally, as we have seen, is to relate all things in ways appropriate to their relations to God. This assumes that something can be known about the relations of things to God, for without such knowledge theological ethics would have no substantive content. This leads to the issues that have elicited the most controversy among Gustafson's critics: the relation between scripture and tradition, experience, and the sciences as sources of this knowledge; the theocentric content these sources yield; and the centrality of nature as clue to the divine ordering.

Gustafson appropriates from the Catholic natural law tradition an emphasis on the importance of nature as a clue to the divine ordering, though with caveats, as we will see. In opposition to most Protestant thought for which God is related to nature through humans, Gustafson mentions with approval Aquinas's belief that humans are related to God, to a significant extent, through the ordering of nature (Gustafson, 1984, p. 44). Gustafson's agreement with this belief extends to its implications for ethics. "The basic pattern of ethics is the right ordering of things in relation to each other as each is related to the other for the sake of the purpose of the whole. And the source for understanding these relations of things to each other is given in the natural ordering of the creation" (Gustafson, 1984, p. 44). Hence a theological construal of nature is of great significance in determining how human beings are to know the divine ordering.

But where does knowledge of the divine ordering come from, what does it tell us, and how does it lead to concrete judgments? It is important to keep in mind what is at stake here. Whether we like it or not, we are faced with the capacities of human beings to increase the scope of their interventions into nature. If the exercise of these capacities ignores the limits of finitude, the requisites of preserving and enhancing human life, and the complex relations of human life to nature (pride), there will be perilous consequences for human beings and for nature itself. Yet human beings by nature and vocation intervene into nature; simply to stop exercising these capacities (sloth) is out of the question. The task of human beings is to participate in the ordering of God, to respond to both the possibilities and limitations it involves. Given the expanded scope and consequences of human action, how we construe this ordering cannot afford wishful thinking or self-serving interpretations.

The problem is that western religious and ethical traditions have always emphasized the utility value of belief for individuals and communities and assured believers that nature and history, or at least the afterlife, ultimately benefit them (Gustafson, 1981, pp. 16–20, 88–95). The problem is exacerbated in the late modern era when religion serves increasingly subjective and temporal ends (Gustafson, 1981, pp. 18–20). Hence, to turn to our major topic, religion can easily be made to legitimate, or at least not to interfere with, the heedless pursuit of relieving the human condition and expanding the range of individual choices that characterizes contemporary medicine. But according to Gustafson, neither experience nor the sciences support the assumption that the cosmos is oriented to the benefit of human beings. To be sure, there are many experiences of human life that support claims about a gracious and loving God, and the biological sciences have unfolded the marvels that gave rise to human life and support it. But there are also painful and tragic experiences that count against the grace and love of God, some of them in the Bible itself, and the sciences speak of the dependence of human beings on nature and of a time when we will no longer be.

This raises the question of the relations between scripture and tradition, experience, and the sciences as sources of knowledge of the divine ordering. In fact these relations are complex and dialectical. For example, there is an irreducible circularity between scripture and experience: scripture itself consists of articulations of a wide range of more general human experiences in light of experiences of God (Gustafson, 1975b, pp. 9–10; 1981, p. 146). Articulation implies language; the experiences of the biblical peoples are inseparable from the symbols, concepts, and genres in which they articulated them.[5] One of the strengths of Gustafson's position is his emphasis on the variety of these articulations of experience, both in terms of genre and plurality of themes. The result is an impatience with efforts to reduce scripture to an overriding theme (e.g., law and gospel or covenant) or a metanarrative (e.g., salvation history). The irony is that while scripture has less authority for Gustafson, he does far less violence to the Bible than do many of his more "biblical" colleagues and critics.

The authority of scripture extends only as far as its interpretations of experience are confirmed in the experiences of the contemporary communities that identify themselves with the biblical peoples. The process is admittedly circular "since the symbols and beliefs of scripture nourish and inform contemporary experience" so that contemporary communities are predisposed to confirm scriptural beliefs, symbols and stories, and their experiences are sufficiently continuous for scripture to have authority. However, the experiences of present communities "are sufficiently discontinuous and different to require other 'authorities' as well" (1975a, p. 161).

This last point sets Gustafson in opposition to those theologians who, while agreeing with him on the dialectical relation of scripture and experience, argue that language is prior to experience in the sense that it does not symbolize independent experiences but rather constitutes a framework that shapes and molds rather than expresses the particular experiences themselves. In George Lindbeck's terms, "theology redescribes reality within the scriptural framework rather than translating Scripture into extrascriptural categories. It is the text, so to speak, which absorbs the world, rather than the world the text" (Lindbeck, 1984, p. 118). Gustafson's claim that the community stands in discontinuity as well as continuity with the biblical tradition is an admission that for him scripture does not absorb the world.[6] This puts the theologian in a complex position vis-à-vis the tradition. It means that he or she stands in continuity with the tradition, but that the tradition is not a sufficient source. One must revise, alter, discard, and add according to persuasive reasons (Gustafson, 1975b, p. 11), and Gustafson has confidence that this can be done responsibly. The theologian for Gustafson is neither formed exclusively by the tradition nor in a neutral standpoint impartially weighing claims from various sources. In Gustafson's own words,

> a theologian can accept accountability for developing aspects of a tradition, being quite explicit about what is discarded from it, how various theological doctrines and principles are recombined as a result of the selection of certain themes to be central, giving reasons for how one works with traditional materials and also rea-

sons for the selection one makes from other ways of explaining and construing the significance of "the world." (Gustafson, 1981, p. 154)

There is no fixed formula for balancing tradition and contemporary experience as sources; in theology as in ethics the exercise of prudential judgment that takes account of the circumstances in which a judgment must be made is decisive.

Of the "other ways of explaining and construing" reality the most prominent for Gustafson are the sciences, especially the biological sciences, though the social sciences also figure strongly. In consistency with his pluralistic use of sources Gustafson does not simply derive theological conclusions from scientific interpretations. But the content of theology can not be incongruous with the data and principles of science (a negative criterion) and must be "indicated" by the latter (a positive criterion) (Gustafson, 1981, p. 257). The sciences—especially geology and evolutionary biology—give no indication that the ultimate purpose of the divine ordering power is the good of human beings (Gustafson, 1981, p. 271). But while Gustafson's major arguments against anthropocentrism are drawn from the sciences, it would be a mistake to suppose that the grounds for theocentrism are purely scientific; he also seeks to recover and highlight neglected theocentric elements in Western religious traditions (Gustafson, 1981, pp. 96–98). His argument involves coherence among a variety of sources.[7]

In conclusion, human experience and the natural and social sciences give descriptions of nature, broadly conceived, and from a theological perspective "the 'ways' of 'nature' are indicators of the ways of God" (Gustafson, 1984, p. 8). Is the theological perspective dispensable? Gustafson argues that one can arrive at the "evaluative descriptions" of nature and humanity summarized in the next few pages from other perspectives (Gustafson, 1981, pp. 3, 15) and he has presented the ethical content of his theocentric perspective without the theology (Gustafson, 1983). However, he is also consistent in arguing that theocentric piety evokes and sustains a conviction of moral significance of the divine ordering and gives some reasons for it (Gustafson, 1981, pp. 3, 15; 1984, pp. 249, 283). This locates piety largely in the realm of motives.[8]

MORAL REASONING AND MORAL CONTENT

Any effort to enlist these sources in the service of concrete moral judgments is bound to be complex, not only because the sources (experience and the sciences) by which theology construes the divine ordering involve perspectival features and require judgments, but also because this ordering itself is complex. Unlike many theologians who look to nature, Gustafson recognizes the ways in which society, culture, institutions, relations between persons, and individual self-determination are inseparable from but not reducible to nature in the strict sense. He also understands that nature is complex, dynamic, and not fully reducible to scientific laws. In what follows I describe four features of "discernment," the process of arriving at particular moral judgments, in relation to four distinct but interrelated claims about nature. For Gustafson, particular moral questions raise questions about what can be discerned about the divine ordering under the circumstances in which they arise.

First, for Gustafson moral discernment identifies points where intervention into a state of affairs is possible. The first task of ethics is to determine "the openings, the occasions, and the interstices in which purposive action is possible" and to locate "the occasions in which the exercise of some capacity or form of power can make a difference to the sequence of events and to the circumstances of the persons involved" (Gustafson, 1975a, p. 11). There are strong echoes of H. Richard Niebuhr's dictum that ethics begins with the question "What is going on?," though Niebuhr's radically situated agent responding to God's actions is replaced by Gustafson's agent facing possibilities of intervening into natural, social and historical processes (Niebuhr, 1963). Both, however, share two important claims: that moral action always occurs in a confluence of factors beyond the agent's direct control though with varying degrees of susceptibility of being shaped by the agent, and that moral analysis is reflection on particular contexts structured by these factors. Interpretation of these factors—the latitude of choice they permit agents, the range of morally relevant features and relations, and so forth—becomes a matter of the first importance.

This view of moral agency and reasoning differs sharply from those that begin with a moral ideal or principle to which they seek to make events and relations conform. Gustafson's argument for his view stresses the rarity of occasions when agents radically initiate action (Gustafson, 1981, p. 333) and points out that even when they do they must take account of an existing course of events and relations in order to be effective in making reality conform to their norms or ends (Gustafson, 1984, p. 9). On these grounds Gustafson regards both abstract moral theories and radical prophetic critiques as insufficient. I return to this point in the conclusion, but here I wish only to stress the importance of the concepts of participation or vocation and of humans as interveners for this view. Moral discernment is carried out by the participant concerned to determine points at which his or her intervention could be effective.

This first point raises the question of the extent of nature's susceptibility to human intervention. Gustafson's reflection on this question bears directly on a major theme of this study: nature for him is not, as Bacon and Locke and their followers have taken it to be, a neutral instrument for the satisfaction of human needs and desires. For Bacon and Locke nature has purely instrumental value. Its destiny is to be subdued by human technology and labor, which by bringing inert nature into an economy of ends rescues it from meaninglessness. For Gustafson nature is not passive or fully subject to human control, and thus is not fully susceptible of being made to serve human ends, including moral ends. Responding to a suggestion by Julian Hartt that he develop a theology of culture, Gustafson replies that were he to do so he would concentrate on human innovativeness in the arts and technology. "With reference to the latter my focus would be on the abiding power of nature to render its 'wrath' on technological activities that are not kept within limits, i.e. on the adverse consequences to life, including human life, from failing to formulate principles of limitation in the control by humans over nature" (Gustafson, 1990c, p. 697).

Two common alternatives to this position are traditional natural law theories and the romantic view of nature shared by the deep ecology movement. What unites these radically different positions is the view that human actions ought to conform to nature. The proper moral stance is resignation. If the view of nature as passive instrument is rendered obsolete by the ever more apparent dangers of human intervention, these latter views are rendered obsolete by the achievements of technology. The traditional natural law position is no longer tenable when human actions themselves can alter nature to the extent that they do. Now "the 'natural order' is less natural in the sense that it is determined simply by 'laws' of nature" (Gustafson, 1984, p. 58).[9] The romantic view of nature must deny the achievements of technology. Gustafson's alternative is to stress participation as "cooperation with nature" (Gustafson, 1981, p. 263) or "consent" to the divine ordering in nature, "a receptivity to possibilities and constraints that exist" (Gustafson, 1983, p. 501). Even medicine, for all its power, must cooperate with nature in order to cure, and nature may at any point resist or deny its efforts, as every physician knows.

This view of nature lends a special moral poignancy to technological interventions. "The moral dimensions of human interventions into nature are located at those junctures where interventions that go 'contrary to nature' or seek to redirect the course of nature are under consideration" (Gustafson, 1981, p. 264). As with Bacon the points of intervention and control of nature are charged with the greatest moral significance, but now it is not because they are the points at which the human condition is relieved or the range of choices is expanded, but because they raise the question of where to draw the fine lines between proper human flourishing and threats to the natural world and to humanity. The simple alternatives of control over nature for human benefit and conformity to nature are replaced by a complex determination of the proper ends, scope and limits of "man the intervener." Once again, it is clear why for Gustafson those engaged in biomedical research are the focus of moral attention, for their interventions into nature explore and test the limits of human cooperation with nature and help determine the proper scope of human well-being. The ideal biomedical researcher is an active participant with nature, preserving and altering its patterns in view of proper ends—a modern and probably secular version of the active Protestant refashioning and reordering the world in accordance with God's will.

Second, as indicated above, a major task of discernment involves an interpretation or "evaluative description" of what is going on (Gustafson, 1981, pp. 333–337). Gustafson has a profound awareness of the role of affections and sensibilities and one's perspective on how one interprets an occasion for moral action. The event or case is always a construction: one makes judgments about what information is relevant, how aspects of the event or case are related, what temporal and spatial range is relevant, how parts are related to wholes, what causal relations obtain. Just as he rejects as an abstraction the imposition of a single principle or set of principles on an event, so Gustafson rejects the notion that there is a single description of an event. He often criticizes bioethics on these grounds, and his criticisms apply to both principlists and casuists (Gustafson, 1981, pp. 329–330; 1987, pp. 36–38).[10] This does not imply that discernment is subjective or relative. One can give reasons for how one describes an event and can account for the choices and sensibilities that shape one's interpretation. One can defend these reasons and choices in conversation with others and can alter them if more persuasive reasons are given. While a rational consensus on moral matters is as unlikely for Gustafson as it is for Aristotle, a community of moral discourse is as necessary for him as it is for Aristotle (Gustafson, 1974, p. 271; 1981, p. 124; 1984, pp. 316–319).

Viewed in light of the chief question of theological ethics, the task of discernment here is to determine how God is ordering various parts in relation to one another and to various wholes. This second claim about discernment brings us to a second claim about nature. According to Gustafson human experiences and various sciences yield strong evidences of human beings and the rest of nature as interdependent. The preservation and well-being of human life and the rest of nature occurs in these "patterns and processes of interdependence": all beings secure their survival and whatever flourishing they achieve only in interaction with others in larger wholes (Gustafson, 1984, pp. 13–19). This claim is closely connected to claims about the good, but the connection is not automatic since values, moral principles and beliefs about the world affect discernments (Gustafson, 1981, pp. 337–338). Hence Gustafson recognizes that it is possible to agree that an adequate description of any entity, event or process must take account of its interdependence in larger wholes while denying the significance of this for ethical judgments (Gustafson, 1984, pp. 14–15). One can argue for example that individual humans are dependent upon larger social and natural wholes but that ethics is concerned only with the rights of individuals or an aggregate of their preferences. Gustafson rejects this ultimately on theological grounds. I will try to reconstruct what I think is his most concise argument. First is a metaethical claim that he borrows from H. Richard Niebuhr without argument: the good is a relational term which must always specify for whom or what something is good (Gustafson, 1981, p. 95; cf. Niebuhr, 1960, pp. 100–109). A descriptive claim follows: human beings are related to other human beings, to institutions, to other living things, and to the biological and chemical conditions of life. A third claim is theological: God governs these patterns and processes of interdependence. The conclusion follows.

> If one's basic theological perception is of a Deity who rules all of creation, and one's basic perception of life in history and nature is one of patterns of interdependence, then the good that God values must be more inclusive than one's normal perceptions of what is good for me, what is good for my community, and even what is good for the human species. (Gustafson, 1981, p. 96)

And if one's moral vocation is to relate all things according to their relations to God, it follows that our moral judgments and actions must take account of larger wholes. This is so not only because the good of the parts depends on attention to the good of larger wholes (though this is generally the case, as Gustafson shows so persuasively in his analysis of marriage and family) but also because the goods of wholes have claims in their own right.

For Gustafson this warrants placing greater weight on the goods of larger wholes and the common good than is found in most moral

theories (Gustafson, 1984, pp. 18–19). Both descriptively and normatively, theocentric ethics takes account of a wider spatial and temporal
frame and larger wholes than other types of ethics. The increased scope
of human action in a technological era and the description of the place
of human beings in the universe given by the sciences expand the range
of morally relevant features (Gustafson, 1983, p. 497) and the perspective of theocentric ethics gives normative status to this expansion. One
result is that the line between obligation and supererogation is not easy
to draw and that consequently self-denial (including self-sacrifice for the
good of others or the common good) may at times be a moral requirement (Gustafson, 1984, pp. 11, 21–22). It would be easy to exaggerate the
significance of this point: in many cases self-denial requires what pru-
dence (enlightened self-interest) would dictate in a theory less concerned with the common good. But Gustafson clearly believes theocentric ethics might involve cases where this happy correspondence would
not hold.

Nevertheless there are several qualifications to this emphasis on
the common good. First, the question of what are the relevant wholes to
be considered depends on what is being considered and the circumstances. After all, as Edward Farley observes, for Gustafson a "whole"
could refer equally to the total ecosystem of the planet, a nation state, or
a hospital (Farley, 1988, p. 41). Discernment involves judgments about
what wholes are relevant to a matter under consideration; it does not
simply apply a formula. Moreover, it is impossible to characterize *the*
all-inclusive whole, and thus impossible to inquire about what is good
for it (Gustafson, 1984, pp. 16–17). Second, theocentric ethics does not
require in every case that the good of a whole take priority over the
good of individuals (Gustafson, 1981, pp. 106, 109; 1984, p. 6). But even
when, as in the case of a doctor deciding whether to perform a costly
procedure on a patient, it is clear that the more limited good of the individual takes priority, one is still required to consider the larger whole so
that it at least becomes harder to justify such actions (though it is not
clear exactly what difference this consideration would make for the
doctor) (Gustafson, 1984, pp. 303–304). Third, Gustafson is aware that
the content of the common good is always defined by those who have
power (Gustafson, 1981, p. 106; 1983, pp. 495–496).

A third feature of discernment is also directly related to a third
claim about nature. Nature changes and exhibits flexibility in the ordering of life. Hence it cannot supply a blueprint for human actions or a
single fixed order of ends and moral principles. Nature changes, due
both to its own development and to human intervention (Gustafson,
1984, pp. 293–294). Human interventions in an age of technology alter

the patterns and processes of interdependence such that moral principles and prohibitions must change. Gustafson's paradigm instance is the capacity of modern medicine and public health to keep people alive longer, thus increasing the population of the planet and requiring once illicit means of population control for the sake of the survival of a larger whole (Gustafson, 1984, pp. 58–60, 228–230). Nature does not order life in a single way. There are certain requisites for human life, for example, or certain parameters to the balance of population and nutritional resources, but they can be met in many ways (Gustafson, 1974, pp. 238–239; 1984, pp. 226–227, 293–294). Moreover, human capacities for self-determination and freedom are themselves part of human nature and limit any efforts to derive a fixed moral order from nature (Gustafson, 1984, pp. 207, 294).

The foregoing features point to a necessary but modest role for claims about nature grounding moral principles and ends. Like Aristotle, Gustafson recognizes that ethics deals with contingent and varying matters so that one can not ask for much certainty. And like Aristotle, Gustafson recognizes that discernment involves perception (cf. Nussbaum, 1986, pp. 264–317; 1990, pp. 54–105) or, in his terms, "an informed intuition" that combines cognitive and affective elements (Gustafson, 1981, p. 338). But Gustafson's position is also grounded in theological claims. He has consistently sought to avoid two extreme positions in his claims about what can be known of the divine ordering. One is the position articulated by Protestants earlier in this century who sought to protect the transcendence of God from idolatrous identifications with merely relative or finite realities. This notion of God is a critical one only; it is devoid of substantive content and thus cannot assist in determining orderings of values and purposes in the finite created order (Gustafson, 1971, pp. 140–141, 143).[11] The second extreme assumes detailed knowledge of God's governance and purposes from reason or revelation or both. Such detailed knowledge would permit the description of a fixed order from which particular moral judgments could be derived or a direct intuition of what God wills or commands in particular contexts.[12]

Gustafson rejects these positions.[13] His alternative argues that provisional knowledge of divine ordering is possible, and that this knowledge is sufficient for many moral judgments though not for moral certainty. For example, one can identify and assign priority to conditions of preservation of life since they have to be met in order for any "higher" purposes to be fulfilled (Gustafson, 1984, pp. 295–298). A strong presumption against taking human life would emerge, on the grounds that physical life is the condition for the realization of any other human values

(Gustafson, 1971, p. 146; 1974, pp. 238–239, 265; 1975a, pp. 46, 157–158). Another presumption in favor of protecting self-determination and for voluntary constraints when constraints are necessary could be defended on similar grounds: self-determination is an important feature of human nature and the condition of the exercise of other capacities as well as a bulwark against tyranny (Gustafson, 1984, pp. 19, 247–248). Hence while human life serves many values which cannot be reduced to a single order and are not always in harmony, we can determine a provisional set of goods and rights that are necessary for the preservation and enhancement of human life, though these may not resolve conflicts in hard cases.[14]

The fourth feature of discernment is its inability to overcome moral conflict and tragedy. "There is no automatic harmony of ideal ends and values; more than one moral principle can make proper claims on conduct, and conflicts between them can not be resolved in all circumstances" (Gustafson, 1984, p. 299). For this reason discernment must take account of the human and other costs of morally justifiable actions. Again, this is directly connected to a fourth claim about the ordering of nature. "God, unfortunately, did not create and does not order all things so that the good of each is in harmony with the good of every other, and even the good of the whole" (1990c, p. 697). This is an early and constant theme of Gustafson's work: meeting the needs or fulfilling the capacities of some family members requires sacrifices even of legitimate needs of other family members and involves tradeoffs between the well-being of individuals and the common good (Gustafson, 1984, pp. 170–172), not all legitimate health care needs can be met (Gustafson, 1984, pp. 273–277), other forms of life are sacrificed for human survival and well-being. In general,

> the legitimate pursuit of legitimate ends, or action in accordance with reasonable moral principles, entails severe losses to others— not only persons but other living things—and even sometimes diminishes the possibilities for development of future life and future generations of human beings. Therein lie the reasons for anger with God. (Gustafson, 1984, p. 21)[15]

Not only is conflict and tragedy between goods often inevitable. There is an even more haunting realization that God does not always order reality such that *any* apparent good is attained. This is often so in the case of human beings: the minimal conditions for physical survival and health are lacking for many people for reasons beyond human control (Gustafson, 1984, pp. 220–221), and sometimes the conditions that enable persons to affirm their lives as worthwhile are altogether lacking (Gustafson, 1984, p. 209). In these and other cases, Gustafson does not flinch: God does not always supply the conditions for human survival and well-being; enmity toward God is the only proper response (Gustafson, 1984, pp. 215–216, 221). But there is also a more general claim. In earlier work Gustafson argued that God's purpose is the well-being of creation (Gustafson, 1975b, pp. 26–36). But in later work he explicitly rejects any Augustinian belief that evils among parts always fit into the good of the whole. While there are grounds for believing that the purposes of the ultimate ordering power are generally good, "the divine governance through nature is not necessarily beneficent. . . . [I]t is not necessarily good for anything or anyone" (Gustafson, 1981, p. 272). This recognition of negation that is not necessarily overcome distinguishes Gustafson from most other theologians is significant for the topic of this volume.

These four claims about nature and their relation to moral reasoning distinguish Gustafson's work from that of others in theological ethics. Gustafson obviously shares with his Protestant and especially Calvinist predecessors a sober, austere, and unromanticized attitude toward nature. One factor in this is his toughminded empiricism that is impatient with claims that ignore or do not cash out in human experiences and practices. Another factor is his strong sensitivity to unrelieved human suffering that is deeply disturbed by efforts (especially religiously sanctioned efforts) to explain away suffering.[16] But in my judgment, both of these elements follow from the ethic of vocation that I believe is central to Gustafson's project. Every ethic of vocation seeks to be effective in the world. For Bacon and the ethic of ordinary life that formed the backdrop to his thought, the mechanization of nature made possible the control over nature that was a condition of effectiveness in serving human needs and glorifying God. Ultimately these processes made possible the technical control over the body that is the basis of scientific medicine. Gustafson's interpretation of nature does something similar for the vocation of responsible intervention. By divesting us of comforting illusions about nature and humanity's place in it and by making us aware of larger wholes, Gustafson hopes to increase our effectiveness in meeting human needs of survival and flourishing while recognizing our limits and the consequences of ignoring these limits. Comforting illusions about nature, often backed theologically by a view of God as ultimately beneficent toward human beings, not only blur the reality of unrelieved suffering, they may also blunt the possibilities that do exist for relieving it. If an ethic of vocation is to be effective in relieving human suffering, it can not afford illusions or false longings about the nature of the world in which that vocation is exercised.

Conditions for relief from human suffering occur; they are dependent upon the patterns of interdependence of life in the world, and ultimately on the divine powers. But they come usually within the confines of the details of life, in the interstices of interaction that enable human intervention to alter the course of events and of individual lives. . . . (Gustafson, 1992a, p. 83)

Gustafson is therefore a realist in two senses: a critical realist who accepts the general reliability of scientific claims about the world and a realist in the anti-utopian sense who focuses on the limits as well as the possibilities of achieving moral and other ends. Both kinds of realism are required by an ethic that is measured by its effectiveness in the world.

PRACTICAL CASUISTRY

In ETP Gustafson treats two issues relevant to bioethics: suicide and allocation of biomedical research funding. In his discussion of suicide Gustafson attempts to overcome traditional treatments of suicide as an act subject to a moral judgment. He appeals to a simple observation: few people today morally condemn persons who commit suicide, and explanations for acts of suicide constitute excusing conditions if not justifications (Gustafson, 1984, p. 187).[17] But Gustafson does not simply exhibit modern sensibility here. Like Karl Barth he believes there is something theologically amiss in moral condemnations of suicide. Such condemnations ignore the reality of what Barth, following Bonhoeffer, called "affliction," and what Gustafson calls "despair."[18]

For Gustafson moral condemnations of suicide focus wrongly on the act itself rather than on the conditions which preserve and sustain life in its interdependence. Such condemnations are wrong in the first place because they assume that persons have capacities to sustain their own lives when in fact these capacities are contingent. As one would expect from Gustafson's descriptions of interdependence, they depend on factors not entirely under the agent's control. It is worth pausing here to note that for both Aquinas and Kant the prohibition against suicide is supported by natural or moral capacities. For Aquinas all persons have a natural inclination to self-preservation so that suicide can be seen as an unnatural act. But Gustafson's awareness of interdependence leads him to emphasize the contingency of the inclination to value life. For Kant, although inclinations contain empirical elements that render them unreliable in establishing the rigorous morality reason requires, the capacity of transcendental freedom enables humans to obey the moral law. But Gustafson's theological commitments prevent him from dismissing the moral significance of natural inclinations and their limitations.

Hence for Gustafson the first task is not to determine the moral rightness or wrongness of particular acts of suicide, since agents do not necessarily have the capacities to act from moral considerations in such cases. Instead the first task is to discern the requisites of the divine governance that enable persons to value their lives and to describe the disorder that occurs when these requisites are not met.

> Interpreted from the perspective of the present work, many suicides follow from, though they are not directly caused by, conditions which cannot be overcome by acts of will based on objective moral arguments. . . . In a sense, then, spiritual or religious factors are involved; there is disorder in the life of the person or in the person's relations to others which leads to despair. (Gustafson, 1984, p. 201)

Gustafson describes the factors constituting this disorder with deep empathy and insight. But whereas Barth is confident that God's grace does address those in despair, Gustafson faces the hard reality that God does not always secure the minimum conditions for persons to affirm their lives as worthwhile. "Alas, for all too many persons there are good and realistic grounds for the deepest despair. . . . To deaths of such persons by suicide one must consent. The powers that bear down upon them are greater than the powers that sustain them. Neither moralists nor God ought to be their judge" (Gustafson, 1984, p. 209). This has serious consequences for theological claims about the benevolence and beneficence of God in particular, and about the capacity of any theology to absorb sorrow and grief. "Finally one has to consent to the reality that the powers that bring life into being do not always sustain it but can lead to its untimely and tragic destruction. No rationalized theodicy or facile assurance of grace removes the pain and the sorrow of the victim and the grieving survivors" (Gustafson, 1984, p. 216).

So far Gustafson has pointed out the limits of moral judgments and theological claims in the face of suicide. He has not yet raised the ethical question, what is God enabling and requiring us to be and do? The short answer is that we are enabled and required "to be participants in the patterns and processes of interdependence that sustain and support the lives of others" (Gustafson, 1984, p. 212). God orders life such that the conditions that enable persons to value their lives are given, when they are given, in interdependence with events, relationships and practices that confer worth on individuals and mitigate despair. In cases where these conditions are threatened the first task of discernment is "to interpret circumstances in light of their alterability"—in other words to identify the "'interstices' in events and relationships and in the history of the self" in which these conditions can be altered (Gustafson, 1984, p. 208). Participation also requires attending to and cultivating those relationships and practices that support and sustain the lives of others. But Gustafson also realizes the limits to human intervention and participation. The self-determination of agents limits what can be done on their behalf, and Gustafson is aware of the destructive consequences of assuming total accountability for the lives of others. Participation is also limited by one's own skill in discerning the conditions needed to avoid despair and in performing the actions needed to secure those conditions, and by the nature of one's relationship to the one considering suicide. Finally, there is no single ordering of the requisites of life that would provide a blueprint for avoiding despair. Sometimes nothing can be done to avoid it.

Only after this broad analysis does Gustafson raise the more narrowly moral question of the justification of particular acts of suicide. The analysis of the act is determined by two claims, one theological and one moral. The theological claim is Barth's dictum that life is no second God; hence its preservation is not an end in itself (Gustafson, 1984, p. 213). The moral claim is that life is of almost absolute value because it is the necessary condition of attaining other values and contributing to others and to larger wholes as a participant, as we discovered above. The almost absolute value of life backs a strong presumption against suicide and an obligation for those who are in a position to do so to restrain persons from commiting suicide. But this presumption can be overridden since physical life is not of absolute value. When unbearable and unrelievable pain and mental anguish are inflicted on persons there is no obligation to endure at all costs, and in cases of refusal of lifesaving medical treatment self-determination must be honored. In both cases, however, justification for overriding the presumption is context-bound: a refusal of treatment by one whose capacity to value life or contribute to others is exhausted is different from a refusal by one whose aspiration for a certain kind of life has been foreclosed by a disabling accident. In the latter kind of case, continuing capacities to value life and contribute to others take priority over a factor such as self-determination that would otherwise justify suicide (Gustafson, 1984, p. 215). But the result is that there are some cases in which suicide must not only be consented to but is also justified. Gustafson, however, is always aware of the loss that occurs even when actions are justifiable. "Suicide is always a tragic moral choice" (Gustafson, 1984, p. 215).

The power of Gustafson's account lies in his deferral of the question of the justification of the act. The deferral of justification is possible because Gustafson's entire account focuses on the capacities of persons to experience the worth and purposes of life for themselves and others. This means that the justification of suicide must consider these capacities rather than more abstract principles such as the sanctity of life or self-determination. Hence Gustafson's account of the value and purpose of physical life avoids the standoff between the absolute value of physical life and the sufficiency of self-determination. It also supplies a criterion for the abatement of medical treatment, though it is not clear who determines when life has lost its value and its capacity to contribute to others or on what grounds. The movement from the contingency of the divine ordering with regard to the capacity to value life to the possibilities and limitations of human participation in that ordering to the question of moral justification places justification in a context that accounts for the whole fabric of our moral lives. By contrast, the poverty of current discussions of physician-assisted suicide by many moral philosophers can be seen in their fixation on self-determination and by their utter neglect of the conditions that lead persons to make a "self-determining choice."[19]

However, one may question whether Gustafson's analysis adequately accounts for the ethos in which assisted suicide and euthanasia are now advocated. The ethos of medicine, as I have argued, is best viewed in terms of Bacon and his successors, with their concern for the relief of the human condition and their confidence that technology allows human lives to be controlled by choice rather than by fate. What is significant is the effort and passion directed toward the control of one's fate at the end of life and the lack of attention to questions of what motivates choices at the end of life. Control is sought for its own sake. There is little room for efforts to discern when life has lost its value for oneself and for others. But questions may be raised about a culture whose idea of freedom is possessing such control for its own sake. Does the necessity of bringing the end of life under the control of human choice constitute a final effort to wrench meaning out of a tragic event in the absence of religious assurances? Does our ability to describe a request for assisted suicide or euthanasia as a choice shield us from a prior abandonment that has driven the patient to her request? Is the effort to control death itself the final expression of a sense of abandonment?[20] The task is to distinguish these situations from those in which decisions follow from convictions about the appropriate limits of pain and suffering, responsibilities to others even in dying, the point at which dignity is irrevocably lost and the conditions under which the inability to derive meaning from an event must be consented to. The point is that the Baconian ethos of medicine is unable make such distinctions. For these convictions depend on a robust view of the ends and purposes of life and the support of others in sustaining them. It is ironic that the very moral theories that profess respect for self-determination and concern for suffering ignore the conditions that force choices and the suffering that results from the abandonment of the ill. But it is also ironic that Gustafson, who recognizes these shortcomings of standard bioethics, fails to say more about what is valued about life and when it is irrevocably lost.

Biomedical research—its nature, limits, and purposes—is the topic of the penultimate chapter of ETP and, as Gustafson notes, it involves all the major themes addressed in ETP (Gustafson, 1984, p. 275).[21] Gustafson's account is governed by the ethics of vocation with its concern for the concrete possibilities and limitations of biomedical research. This means, first, that he takes the standpoint of the engaged participant rather than that of the disengaged moral theorist or the prophetic critic. I criticize this distinction below, but its implications are clear. "The ethical task is to contribute to the direction of events that are taking place" (Gustafson, 1984, p. 271). The type of moral discourse involved is therefore policy discourse, which differs from ethical or prophetic discourse. Whereas the "ethical observer" begins with the question of what ought to be the case, the "engaged agent" begins with the question of what is possible (Gustafson, 1990b, p. 140). Hence much of Gustafson's account is descriptive; it attempts to map the various interacting processes that bear upon biomedical research and to locate points of possible intervention. "One has to be able to interpret what is going on in order to know at what points intentional interventions do and can occur, and thus at what points some possible alteration of a course of events can be made if that is desirable" (Gustafson, 1984, p. 255). Gustafson considers several of these courses of events: the politics of various interest groups, the administration of scientific research, the various circumstances of individual researchers, and the processes of carrying out research and distributing its results. He also describes the medical, ethical, economic, and political criteria that in fact govern biomedical research funding.

But this does not mean that ethical arguments are unimportant, since one needs to know what kinds of interventions into these courses of events are desirable. Ethical argument "articulates ends, refines the criteria for the moral choices embedded in the empirical, and facilitates moral self-evaluation" (Gustafson, 1990b, p. 141). Accordingly, Gustafson